C000088958

SPLENDOR

The Nazarite Method to Re(growing) Long, Strong, Healthy, Holy Hair

Sara Sophia Eisenman

Copyright © 2018 Sara Sophia Eisenman
All rights reserved.

Cover art by: Sara Sophia Eisenman
Photos by: Hanan Eisenman

ISBN: 1-7901-2616-9
ISBN 13: 9781790126163

TABLE OF CONTENTS

INTRODUCTION:
Will This Method Work For Me If...?

A warm hello and thank you for reading *Splendor: the Nazarite Method to (Re)growing Long, Strong, Healthy, Holy Hair*. In 2016 at the age of 40, I experienced dramatic hair loss generated by stress and trauma (coupled with physical factors such as changing hormones), which left me with a large bald spot on the back of my head and dramatic thinning overall.

This personal crisis led me on a deep quest to deepen and expand my already-existing work on healing trauma in the body to more fully understand hair, its special needs and functions, and how to generate optimal health in hair for myself and others. As a result of this intense and experiential quest, my hair loss not only fully, miraculously healed, but also far transcended its previous maximum length and health, exceeding my own expectations of the possible.

At age 43 as of my birthday tomorrow, the bald spots have completely filled in and my hair is now longer, thicker, stronger and shinier than its ever been in my entire life, even as I "should" (according to society's views) be starting to decline due to age. Thus, on the eve of my 43rd birthday, I am having a blast feeling the healthiest and most vital that I've ever been in my entire life, and sporting ever-longer silver mermaid locks to boot, which - divine be willing - will soon reach waist-length. I am so excited to share all the wisdom that I've uncovered along this path with you, to help you create a practice of hair re(growth) grounded in real results, and to support you in your own journey with strong, healthy hair every step of the way!

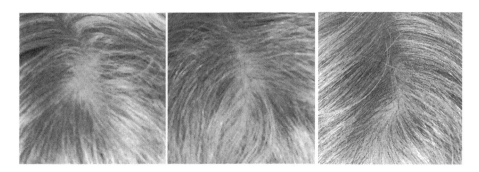

Above: Unretouched images of the back of my head at three different points in my recovery, in approximately November 2016, July 2017, and September 2017, respectively. I had developed a noticeable bald spot that filled in completely, in addition to filling in areas at the temples and along the hairline that had exhibited thinning, as well as thickening and strengthening of the hair overall using the Nazarite method.

The method I have developed as a result of my own recovery from hair loss - in partnership with my amazing husband and gifted shaman Hanan who has been key in creating and implementing this healing process for and with me - is holistic and comprehensive: spanning energetic, nutritional, supplemental and topical care. It is actually a full-body, full-being means of healing; and if employed, will almost surely benefit not only the hair but one's life in total. In the understanding of the method I am about to outline, our hair is not treated as separate or isolated from the total self, but rather honored fully in the context of the whole and particularly in its function as a sacred antenna and conduit of information and power, which connects profoundly with the nervous system and the body's innate knowing. As such, our hair becomes fully honored in a beautiful, potent, meaningful practice as we establish a real way of working with the power of the hair, intentionally cultivating its health through intention and dedication.

It's important for me to state at the outset that I am not a hair "expert" per se, nor a medical doctor, nor have I conducted controlled scientific studies on this method and its outcomes. This protocol is not designated in any way as a substitute for medical care, and specific potential physical conditions correlating/corresponding to hair loss are discussed more below that the reader may be informed and deeply consider what all is relevant to them, and continue to seek appropriate care and support accordingly.

However, what I *can* tell you is that I have dedicated my entire life to a deep - as yet perhaps rare - understanding and embodiment of energy and its functioning in our living systems as human beings, and that there are very few physical conditions - including hair loss - that will not respond highly positively to, if not be fully resolved by, deep energetic understanding and care. It is from this perspective that I feel qualified to speak to the sanctity of this method and its potential for efficacy across a wide swath of individuals and situations.

I also feel confident in saying that this is a "do no harm" sort of method, and that - in addition to its potential to help regrow hair - it also can and will only result in improvement of total health overall, particularly since each individual's discernment (in the form of their real-time relationship with their own body and knowing), is absolutely honored and built-in at every turn. As such, I want to re-emphasize at this turn that one is strongly encouraged to never go against one's own deep knowing in using *any* healing practice, whether this or any other; and to take/use only that which applies to and honors oneself. Developing your own relationship with your unique body, and honoring its needs, is absolutely paramount to this and *all* healing processes.

It is also important to note that when you undertake the work introduced in this book, what arises as a result may ask you to change not only your diet and the grooming habits and care regarding your hair specifically, but possibly even your life: in ways including but not limited to resetting your personal boundaries, breaking addictions, speaking difficult truths, severing ties with unaligned people, places and things, and undertaking notable personal transformation. This was certainly, absolutely, inescapably true in my case.

At this point you may be thinking, "All I want to do is regrow my hair, not change my entire life!" But, our hair can be understood as both a vital, living record of our energy and the antenna through which we exchange vast amounts of energy and information, perhaps even more than our other senses. Understood at this depth, it makes sense that it can only be healed in the context of caring for the total self *and* that there is a profound reclamation on offer.

Of course, it could be argued that there are much "easier" ways to (re)grow your hair - take this magic pill, use this wonder shampoo! - yet many of these will be either an ineffectual waste of time or a cosmetic, bandaid solution. This is in marked contrast to getting to the crux of the matter and working from there, non-invasively, with no use of chemicals and procedures - strictly from the inside out in a thorough and rigorous way - as does the method of this book. In addition, if one addresses only one aspect and not others (say, topical care but not nutrition, or nutrition without energy considerations), then there is a lower probability of seeing results - whereas a more comprehensive method holds the best and highest chance of seeing results quickly and for all the right reasons. Because of this, I

4

recommend implementing the entire method (or as much as you truly can), in order to see the best, most lasting and real results.

In light of all of this, and of your specific concerns, you may be asking before we begin: *but will this method work for me?* The answer is that we are all individual and many factors are in play, so results will inevitably vary - that said, this method has a great deal of potential to help people from all walks of life. Whether you are simply seeking to grow longer, stronger hair; are recovering from chemotherapy or other medical treatments; are a man with male-pattern hair loss seeking regrowth; are a woman with hormonal changes and health factors affecting your hair, etc. - this method offers deep and real practical considerations and means of recovery. I address each of these questions in more detail, here:

-Can this help me if I am a cancer survivor and have lost hair/hair changes due to chemotherapy?

Yes, it can. This will greatly assist your regrowth process and is also supportive for recovery for the entire body and being following aggressive medical treatments such as chemotherapy. In this case, I strongly recommend a great deal of nutritional replenishment and nurturance, in addition to energetic/ shamanic work, to nourish yourself amply, help restore excellent cell health and functioning and also to restore a feeling of safety and trust in the entire body, which extends to the hair. Specific practices, such as veiling the hair for a time, may be tremendously beneficial in these cases.

-Can this help me if I am a man with male-pattern baldness?

Again, yes. For men, an emphasis is placed upon the detoxification and shamanic/energetic aspects of this method (explained in much more detail in the following sections) - as the cells/follicles may have become damaged or deactivated due to hormones acting upon them. However, given persistence and faithful application of this method in total, male pattern baldness can indeed be significantly improved or even totally reversed naturally. My husband Hanan is now in the process of regrowing his own male-pattern hair loss and is seeing significant regrowth. We feel confident that many others will follow suit and see improved results in hair growth.

-Can this help me (re)grow my hair if I'm still coloring/dyeing?

The answer is yes, it will likely still help; but it is not recommended as optimal for full recovery if you are experiencing hair loss. As mentioned above, the hair is a very sensitive, sacred antenna of the nervous system and is literally designed to receive, store, and exchange energy in such a way as to impart wellness to the entire body - while reflecting that wellness in the form of its own vitality and shine. When it is artificially coated with chemical dyes, it is difficult for this process of receiving and metabolizing light/information to take place in its natural form, and the chemicals themselves are mostly toxic to hair cells and follicles - sometimes dangerously so - inhibiting proper function.

If you do choose to continue dyeing (for which there is absolutely no judgment as I myself colored my hair for fifteen years!), you will likely still see positive results, and/but the results will be enhanced by taking the step of freeing the hair of dyes. Henna and other natural dyes may be an exception to this rule and should be discerned on a case-by-case basis - but in any case if you are experiencing extreme hair loss and wishing to reverse this, I strongly encourage you to forego even natural dyes for a time until your hair has fully recovered, and from there, reassess your needs and desires in this regard (as you may well decide you don't want or need the hair color after all!).

If you are planning to transition to natural silver hair as a part of this protocol and would like community in this, please be invited to join our group *The Silver Circle* on Facebook, which is designed to support and inspire people in precisely this process and help everyone feel beautiful as their natural dye-free self, and is currently several thousand wonderful members strong.

-Can this still help me regrow my hair if I am vegan and therefore cannot utilize the non-vegan aspects of the protocol?

Again, yes, there will be benefits but I cannot guarantee maximum gains from this approach, and this will tend to vary greatly from person to person. Although not agreed upon by all, I personally have found that - particularly for menstruating women and people with certain constitutions and body types - certain animal-based foods can be very nourishing for people experiencing hair loss and a host of other conditions. This is not to say one cannot be optimally healthy as a vegan, and I certainly admire and understand the impetus to want to spare animals any suffering and eat vegan. Yet in my own duty to speak truth to my personal experience in working with myself and others, I have found that sometimes well-sourced animal foods such as cod liver oil, bone broths etc. are key to rapid healing and nutrient replenishment - and upon total recovery, consumption of animal foods may be carefully modified/

minimized or even eliminated in many cases while optimal health is retained. Animal foods are a small, yet in some cases, quite vital aspect of this protocol; and if you are a vegan experiencing notable hair loss, you may wish to consider if diet is playing a role in overall health. That said, the other aspects of the protocol will surely bring benefits and are well worth exploring and implementing. In several areas of this book, I have added additional recommendations for vegans or substitute means of obtaining certain key nutrients.

Lastly - and perhaps most importantly - as you read this book and begin to implement the method as you choose, please don't sweat *any* of it in a way that feels stressful. Just do the best you can, learn as you go, stay in the productive zone where you are challenging yourself to practice the best self care possible but also giving yourself grace, and trust that it's perfect. Also, even if you do every single thing "right" (which is completely unique to each person), it can take a matter of six months to a year to even really *begin* to see the results that are possible. Please keep this in mind and commit to stay the course without fixating on "results" for at least six months. Just keep nourishing yourself and refining and deepening as you go.

In my own process, I definitely made some errors (such as an overaggressive massage that made my bald patch worse before it actually got better), and also at times lost faith and became depressed, slacked off and "cheated" on certain aspects when I was too tired, didn't remember, was in resistance, or had other priorities that I had to tend to first. Rather than get discouraged or become self-judgmental, I kept going. And over the long haul, my hair not only regrew but is now way better than ever before; and yours can be too! Just do the best you can, hang in there, and stay in the mindset and heartset of gentle confidence, belief in yourself, patience, and above all self-love.

In addition to the information and support offered in this book, we have created a few other offerings specifically designed to support you in your hair growth journey, ranging from an online hair group so you can meet and share experiences and information with other like-minded individuals as you utilize the method in this book, to energy work facilitated by my husband Hanan Eisenman that "diagnoses" the deep causes of hair loss and generates regrowth on the deepest energetic level, to a special consulting session in which I create a custom hair growth plan with/for you and send a full report with your detailed recommendations. More information about these offerings can currently be found at my website www.sarasophiaeisenman.com. I hope you will utilize these additional tools as you feel called, as wonderful ways to engage the Nazarite method contained in this text as fully as possible for yourself and generate amazing results!

CHAPTER 1: *More of My Hairstory & What is the Nazarite Method?*

The Nazarite method is a means of regrowing hair developed by my ever fuller understanding of the true nature of hair as alive, energetically important, and highly responsive to our inmost beings, sense of self, and use of our life force. Many traditional cultures have known for millennia that our hair is not "dead" at all - as lots of Western "experts" claim - but rather functions as an antenna for energy and a literal extension of the nervous system.

As a receiver of information, our hair is most alive indeed, and can and will reflect the state of our overall being and the frequencies/dynamics to which we are attuned. Much like a radio tower can be attuned to different frequencies aka "stations," so too can our hair - and some frequencies are much more health-promoting and sustaining than others in this regard. Because of the sensitivity of our hair, it can "pick up" and function as a conduit for the energies of any unaligned dynamics in our life that are not serving us in the highest, and will then reflect these dynamics in its overall health and appearance. Our hair also contains our history, as - like the layers of an archeological site revealing details of whole civilizations - its layers hold many details about our diet, our stress levels, our reproductive histories, even our relationships, at various points in time.

In my own interesting journey with my hair, I have had the opportunity to discover this wisdom firsthand. My first inkling that hair is energetically alive and powerful came at just 21 years of age, when - in going through a spontaneous rite of passage and processing much of the trauma of my difficult childhood - my hair turned from its original dark brown color to completely silver, literally overnight.

I remember being absolutely horrified as I peered at my roots in the mirror and suddenly saw sprouting from all over my head the all-too conspicuous silver roots that I associated much more with my mother than myself. My mom had also gone gray early too, and had a very unhappy relationship with her hair - lacking the money to color it regularly and feeling ashamed of and stigmatized by her silver locks. Calling herself names like "ugly" and "old." Wishing she had the means to disguise it. Sometimes she simply wouldn't raise her head in public, despite the objective fact that she was/is quite beautiful.

Determined not to suffer a similar fate, I began coloring my hair every two to three weeks from that tender age of 21, frantic to cover the "evidence" of my silver and keep it that way! My hair grows extremely fast and the roots were nearly always peeking out - so I spent a great deal of time feeling ashamed, covering my head with hats and headbands to conceal either the tell-tale ring of black chemical stain left on my skin after coloring, or the annoying gray that would inevitably become visible almost as soon as I could "get rid" of it. I even used a plethora of toxic, messy products to try and blend the roots, such as hair "crayons" or powders made of who-knows-what, often with disastrous and simply gross results.

And so it continued, for about 15 years, through college, work, marriage, and two children. This "secret" I was always trying to keep was such an ingrained part of my everyday existence that the strong negative emotions I held with regards to my hair and myself became almost subliminal, pushed deeply into my unconscious so I could pretend it didn't matter. There were times that I turned down invitations from friends because my roots were showing or - like my mother - that I could not raise my head or look others squarely in the eye because I was ashamed of my gray. Yet all of this remained somehow below the surface as I carried on "as usual."

As a busy mom and writer in my 30's, it suddenly occurred to me how utterly bizarre it is that so many of us feel compelled to disguise our true hair in order to feel beautiful or accepted by society, not to mention the undesirability of the massive toxic load of dye and shame constantly being heaped upon my own head. I quickly began to realize it was one thing to choose to color my hair, but quite another to feel *less* than OK for choosing not to.

I started to ponder the question: what was so very wrong with my gray that I must continuously cover it? The layers of shame and unprocessed emotion associated with my hair began to surface, and as I "unpacked" these layers, I was delighted to arrive at the following revelation: There was nothing at all "wrong" with me or my hair!

As I began my transition, I came to see my shiny silver roots as beautiful: an exquisite and profound symbol of the divine feminine, not ugly or shameful at all. I stopped looking at myself and all my "flaws" with harsh judgment – which I wasn't even fully consciously aware of doing in the first place – and instead, began to look at myself with softer, more accepting gaze. This new self-acceptance applied not only to my hair but also to all that I am. I realized that holding myself to the standard of society's narrow and actually quite violent version of "beauty" (or at least to the way I interpreted that standard) had been holding me back from developing and stepping out with other parts of myself – my intellect, my compassion, my wisdom. Suffice it to say, my transition was literally revelatory and taught me an enormous amount about what all was "hiding" underneath that dye - and it wasn't just silver hair!

As my hair grew, I found it created quite a stir everywhere I went. People who held false expectations as to who I was "supposed" to be became critical of my decision and fell to the wayside in my life, and I was met with much more open-minded and interesting people. And to my amazement, people everywhere from the grocery store to my kids' park to Facebook would often get so excited and inspired by my silver that they soon embarked upon their own journeys to embracing their natural hair, and began sending me notes of thanks via social media from all over the world!

From all of this, I began to develop a knowing that there is something very special about hair; it is not just this dead stuff that sprouts from our heads as modern biology would have us believe, but something much more potent than that: a magical living crown that has the power to activate ourselves and others, to cultivate magic, to receive and embody wisdom; and much more.

Proverbs 16:31 of the Hebrew bible encodes this knowing, specifically with regards to gray hair, stating, "Gray hair is a crown of splendor; it is attained in the way of righteousness." Working with many silver haired men and women since then, I have found this to very often be true - there is a great correspondence between spiritual/shamanic trials and silvering of the hair. There are (as with all things) at least two ways to look at this: one is that we are "aging" or somehow "declining" in beauty and vitality; and another is that we are attaining wisdom through trial by fire, initiation and choosing to rise. One thing

I've learned well from my own experience and that of many others is that silver hair is not necessarily a function of age; it very often is a function of *experience*, and thereby, wisdom. As such, it is actually a marker of a beautiful, special, regal sort of power that is much needed at a time when wisdom can save us. This important re-frame of silver hair is part of the work I'm so excited and grateful to perform in the world, helping people everywhere to see that their silver hair *is* splendid and beautiful - a crown indeed - and even to watch young people aspire to "earn" their own silver through walking the way of wisdom, beauty and righteousness.

However, despite a burgeoning understanding of the power and value of silver hair, at this juncture of my journey I still did not have all the pieces to this puzzle nor was yet living them in an embodied way. I still took my hair and its health largely for granted, expected it to simply grow and "perform" as I wanted it to without the requisite nurturance and care or much consideration at all, and held quite a great deal of unconscious violence toward myself and my hair not being "good enough," a deep lack of self-worth that I tried to compensate for by trading on my hair/looks, etc. This is the plight of so many of us, particularly women who are learned to view our hair/looks as a social currency rather than an inherently sacred part of who we are.

But soon enough, my hairstory encountered another major plot twist, as in 2016 I went through a very difficult, painful experience - another shamanic initiation of sorts - and my hair began falling out in handfuls, leaving me with bald spots (per the photos shown earlier) and increasing despair. Having worked so hard to grow out my silver hair and seeking to grow long mermaid locks to my waist, this loss was devastating to me and I had to cut my hair short to deal with the sad mess left on my head.

To make a very long story short, at this time my hair was massively infiltrated by unaligned and destructive energies, as dynamics of childhood abuse - which I had suppressed - painfully resurfaced in a destabilizing and endangering manner and were opportunistically seized upon by some parties interested in using them to their own advantage, to put it mildly. I was caught in the "spin cycle" of this situation for the better part of a year before I finally found a way through it, much worse for the wear and having lost a great deal of hair in the process. A huge part of the real-time resolution of this situation and its accompanying hair loss - which threatened not only my hair but my health and life overall - was to revoke the access of *ALL* unaligned energies and dynamics with regards to my hair (and by extension, to my total self), while rededicating my hair and myself to healthy, whole, loving, sustaining dynamics that would allow for complete recovery and healing. This process was combined with and supported by excellent, constitutionally-aligned nutrition and topical hair care.

The total protocol, which I have been implementing ever more fully for the last one and a half years' time, has resulted in astounding revelation, miracles and health; and I am still deepening my relationship with it and learning more each and every day. You can see the results of devoted application of this method in the photos below, spaced just a single year apart. The photo on the left was taken on my birthday in September 2017 (hence the fancy birthday crown), while the photo on the right is September 2018. By this time my bald spots had already primarily filled in, and I experienced a continuing increase in thickness as well as rapid growth in that single year, surpassing my longest length with no signs of slowing.

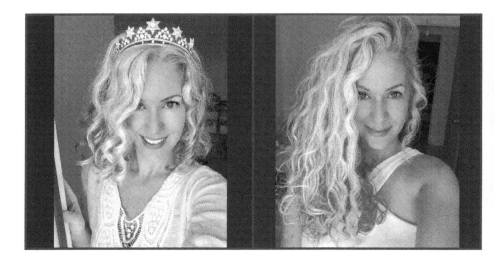

And that is how the Nazarite method of hair regrowth, as I have come to call it, was born into my life. The concept of the Nazarite - for those who are not yet familiar - comes from the Hebrew bible, to describe one who has voluntarily taken a vow to separate him- or herself as holy, as described in Numbers 6.[1] Indeed the word "Nazarite" comes from the Hebrew word *nazir* meaning "consecrated" or "separated," which denotes being set apart for the divine, as one's being becomes a designated, sacred receiver and container of purposeful and well-directed energy. Because hair is understood in this ancient context as a sacred and powerful receiver and embodiment of energy - both an extension of the nervous system and a conduit of divine power - the Nazarite oath detailed in Numbers very specifically articulates that the hair in particular be grown long in devotion, and then dedicated very specifically to the Divine if/when finally cut it, as the culmination of the oath.

---

[1] See Appendix A at the back of this book for the full text describing the Nazarite oath, as articulated in Numbers in the Hebrew bible.

In my own modern-day and relatively non-religious translation of this Nazarite oath, I have dedicated my hair as an antenna *only* of the highest good, and abstained from cutting my hair except for a once yearly option to trim (which I actually have not elected to do yet, now more than 1.5 years into the process). When I do finally trim my hair, the clippings will be saved and devoted intentionally to a divine altar - either by being buried and thereby returned to the Earth, or by being burned and therefore sent as a smoke offering to the Sky. This set of commitments can of course be customized to your individual needs and desires, and may not look the same as mine (remember this is far less about religious rules than it is about finding your own true north) - but the basic principles of: 1) dedicating one's hair to the highest good through specific practices, and 2) returning trimmed or clipped hair to nature through intentional means, are core to this method as intentional forms of energetic hygiene and cultivation of aligned power, in ways that we will explore together shortly.

Somewhat relatedly, it is also detailed in Numbers that to be a Nazarite, one must abstain from intoxication in the form of alchoholic drink (specified as wine). For me in the modern-day context, this translates to a commitment to eliminate intoxicating and addictive patterns and habits in my own life - not only in the form of alchohol but in the form of *anything* potentially destructive, compulsive and habit-forming - to cultivate freedom of choice and discipline that allows me to abstain at will from anything habit-forming, and most importantly to generate ecstacy and joy from a place of absolute clarity, acute devotion and sobriety, which as it happens is the best and truest "high" of all. Again, this is core to the method described in this book in ways that will become clear in a moment - notably through a weekly protocol involving one's hair that will be used to purify/

cleanse all addiction and devote/return one's energy to one's own full alignment and "true north" - outlined fully in the next chapter.

The Nazarite passage in Numbers then concludes with a blessing, intimating that anyone who chooses to devote themselves in this way will be gazed upon by the Divine countenance in favor and splendor, abundantly bringing blessings not only upon him- or herself, but that all the people will benefit because of the righteous relationship with themselves and the Divine that has been undertaken, and to which the Nazarite fully commits.

The reason for this resulting vitality and bountiful blessing is a matter of natural, energetic law that can be understood in terms of circuitry. The human being is essentially an energy circuit - with the hair being a, if not *the*, primary antenna of the entire system. When the circuit is broken, the hair is then available to energies that use and siphon the system, creating an energetic scenario in which life force is continuously leaking out and/or being drained in a power reversal - and the circuit thus consistently experiences a net loss of vitality. But when the circuit is reclaimed, cleansed, rededicated and amply nourished by being attuned to the sacred frequencies that nurture instead of draining - it then completes itself, creating a self-sustaining dynamic that is more than the sum of its parts. There is a very practical and simple way of doing this that can make an unbelievable difference in your hair and your entire life.

The way this practice works in my life - and can work for you also - does not necessarily involve adherence to a specific religion in a dogmatic sense, and can be understood purely in terms of energy usage and natural law. That said, there is a beautiful sense of divine splendor, awe and recognition of miracles that does arise as a natural result of adhering to this protocol that one can only describe as an experience of something transcendent and beyond one's finite human self. In a funny way, the experience of overflowing joy and vitality can be seen as just another wonderful "side effect" of the practice of having fantastic hair! These do indeed co-occur. However you personally choose to view it, this practice of devotion has glorious benefits all the way around, which overflow to all.

And now: enough with the theory and abstract talk, let's get to some details of healing and growing that hair!

CHAPTER 2: *Hair Loss, Root Cause Concerns & Considerations*

While not completely comprehensive, this chapter is offered as a brief overview of some things that can cause hair loss and some ways to begin addressing these. The method that I will outline in detail in the following chapters will be beneficial for nearly all of them, and it's also good to be aware of the various factors in play so that you can better glean where you stand with each of them and place the emphasis where it's most needed.

As described in the last chapter, I feel that my hair loss in 2016 stemmed primarily from energetic infiltration, and stress/trauma are indeed primary causes of hair loss. Energetic and trauma-based infiltration of the hair can come in many forms, including acute traumas, codependent or addictive relationships, stressful or unaligned work environments, substance abuse habits, internet/technology overusage and really any other major stressor or addiction. This can also include any negative/low worth beliefs that we unconsciously hold about ourselves/our health/our hair, based on what we were told or how we were treated in childhood. These destructive dynamics and patterns of infiltration can be tricky and difficult to spot, having become "part of us" in a way that makes them nearly invisible until we finally unearth and clear them. In employing this method, you will have a chance to quite literally wash these dynamics rite out of your hair (remember the old song?), while introducing and sealing in those energies which are nurturing, healing and committed to wholeness.

Chronic stress, in particular, is something that must be addressed and lifestyle changes made to minimize it for optimal health not only of our hair, but our total beings. Hair is exquisitely sensitive and registers everything that is going on with us energetically. Meanwhile, many of us are living day-to-day existences mired in stress that keep our cortisol levels elevated and our adrenals pushed to the max, resulting in fatigue and auto-immune issues. It may be necessary, to restore your health and hair, to assess where in your life stress is playing a role and what can be done to prevent, or at the very least, regularly detoxify stress chemicals from your system and return to a more relaxed homeostatis. Time in nature, regular bathing protocols, a peaceful working environment, a regular mindful/ spiritual practice, and loving relationships are important keys to working to release your stress in positive ways. To this end, ritual/ceremonial bathing has become a very important practice in my life and a key part of the Nazarite method, as you will see shortly; and has actually helped to regrow my hair.

Another primary cause of hair loss is malnutrition or chaos in the body caused by a high-inflammatory, low nutrient diet. It's no secret that the standard American diet (SAD) generates a huge amount of toxicity in our systems, which can have a tremendous effect on our hair. Many Americans, even when we think we are eating a "healthy" diet, end up malnourished in various categories due to poor soil and growing conditions and other factors, while ingesting too much sugar and refined/artificial foods that completely confuse the body and lead to suboptimal health. The next chapter of this book is devoted solely to nutritional considerations that can affect the hair and how to make sure we are getting enough of what we need, while minimizing what is not beneficial.

There can also be a multitude of physical factors and correlates that affect hair health, including but not limited to: thyroid conditions; anemia; autoimmune issues; shifting hormones due to pregnancy, loss of pregnancy, peri-menopause and menopause; and primarily for men, testosterone in its action upon the hair follicles.

Most of these physical conditions can actually be healed and their effects upon hair mitigated and even reversed completely through the protocol outlined in this book, particularly when shamanic journeywork is included to really kick-start the healing process. As I will detail further in the chapters detailing the three phases of the protocol, the healing shamanic journeywork offered by my husband Hanan has been absolutely instrumental in helping to heal and restore my hair, and is a great boon to this protocol. Not only does it have a huge capacity to clear and reset the energetics of the hair, it also helps to heal physical illnesses and/or causes of hair loss at the very root of the issue, as has been the case for many of Hanan's clients. (This healing capacity applies to all physical illness, not only ones that affect hair.)

If you feel you are experiencing significant health challenges that are affecting your hair, consider employing this healing modality along with any/all others that support your total health. For a more detailed explanation of how and why shamanism (and in particular the shamanism that Hanan practices) works so effectively to resolve physical illness, you can dive into our recent book *God is with Us: A Manual of Journeys* and read detailed information about the practice, as well as case studies of how it's helped so many to achieve full-being healing. For now, we turn - in the next chapters - to the specifics of proper nutrition, and then to the three phases of the Nazarite method in detail.

CHAPTER 3: *On Nutrition - What You Need to Know for Healthy Hair*

Many nutrients, both micro and macro, are needed to support healthy hair growth. We will visit each of these in this chapter and provide a sample day's nutrition to support you in being amply nourished for your journey to optimal hair health. In addition, for balanced health overall, it's really important that you assess your own constitution at this time and eat according to your specific needs as well as your unique health history. I will provide some basic tools to get you started with this, and the rest will be a process of listening closely to your body and fine-tuning your own relationship with nutrition accordingly. Excellent nutrition will provide the ideal foundation to ensure that the three phases of the protocol have the very best chance of succeeding as your hair heals, so you can start right away with this (even today, before you read the rest of the book!), and use this information to nourish yourself and your hair throughout the entire process.

In order to grow strong and healthy, hair needs ample proteins including a full range of amino acids, good fats and fatty acids, and a wide range of nutrients including zinc, copper, selenium, vitamin D, vitamin A, iron, silica, B vitamins, vitamin C, vitamin E, and more. In general, it's best to get these nutrients in real food sources as opposed to popping a bunch of supplements, for a couple of reasons: 1) supplements tend to be less fresh/bioavailable, therefore poorly absorbed, and don't always contain what they say they do - so you don't really know what you are getting in terms of actual usable nutrition. 2) Certain nutrients are necessary to have in correct amounts and ratios, and having too much is just as toxic as having too little. Nature tends to supply these nutrients in ratios that our bodies can use in balance and synergy, preventing us from OD-ing on one while having too little of another; while supplements can tend to easily throw these ratios off balance.

That said, it's fine to use a few supplements in moderation and to balance out your nutrient profile (I do!); just make sure that you are getting the bulk of your nutrition from fresh, whole, organic/wild sourced foods to the greatest extent possible, and that any supplements you employ are high quality and ideally food-sourced (as opposed to synthetic). The few supplements that I use/recommend will be listed in this chapter and you can always experiment with your own; just do your research and use discernment, as you don't want to throw off the total balance or add toxicity.

Foods and supplements that I have found especially good for nourishing and regrowing hair (with my very favorites at the top), include:

-well sourced (wild) salmon and seafood such as shrimp, crab, and oysters: *contains key nutrients including zinc, copper and selenium*
-black currants and black currant oil (taken as a supplement): *contains beneficial fatty acids, anti-inflammatory; balances hormones*
-fish oil and/or fermented cod liver oil: *contains essential fatty acids excellent for hair and nervous system, cod liver oil contains ample vitamins A & D in the correct ratios*
-avocados: *amazing hair and skin superfood containing healthy fats, fatty acids, vitamins B, E and more*

-spirulina: *incredibly high in protein and amino acids, B vitamins, copper and iron*

-pomegranate juice: *the seeds contain punicic acid that strengthens hair follicles and promotes circulation; also contains tons of antioxidants*

-carrots and carrot juice: *high quantity of vitamins including beta carotene, which translates in the body to vitamin A*

-garlic: *potent anti-bacterial and anti-fungal that helps detox the whole body, reset microflora balance and strengthen the immune system*

-bone broth: *contains many necessary ingredients for hair and connective tissue, including proteins and needed minerals*

-collagen powders: *contains proteins responsible for maintaining the strength and elasticity of nails, skin and hair*

-eggs: *densely packed with nutrition and proteins, including biotin, folate, vitamin A and D; can be taken/added to smoothies raw if you have an extremely fresh, pastured, organic source*

-most all nuts and seeds, especially pepitas (pumpkin seeds): *contains fats, fatty acids, protein; pepitas contain high iron, zinc and copper*

-leafy greens: *high in antioxidants and iron*

-hemp seeds: *high in helpful proteins and good fats*

-berries of all varieties: *power-packed with antioxidants*

-horsetail and nettles (taken together as a tea): *great source of silica and iron; nettles regulate hormones*

-red meat/organ meat as supportive to boost nutrient supply/reverse anemia: *this is like a hard-core multi-vitamin if you have lost blood through heavy periods or have become malnourished over time*

Further elaborating on the above, I actually have found a couple of supplements quite useful - including a hair multi-vitamin called Viviscal, which contains vitamin C, niacin, biotin, calcium, iron and zinc, along with horsetail, millet extract and a patented "aminomar" blend of oyster powder and shark cartilage. While one could source these same nutrients in a food-based manner, it's helpful to have them all in one place and I've never experienced a negative effect from this product. I also supplement with fish oil and/or fermented cod liver oil, black currant oil (as capsule form is nearly the only way to get this oil in the US), and pomegranate extract in capsule form. These supplements and all other supplement-type products that I use are listed in Appendix B, for your ease of reference.

Just as important as eating the right foods, is making sure you are not eating the *wrong* ones. Foods and substances that are not generally helpful for healthy hair growth - or health in general - include: white sugar, cigarettes/habitual tobacco use, anything artificial, partially hydrogenated or easy-rancidified oils, processed corn products such as high fructose corn syrup, unfermented soy, refined white grains, monosodium glutamate or other additives that affect the nervous system, pesticide-laden or GMO fruits and vegetables, and factory-farmed/processed meats or dairy. All of these acidify the body, promote inflammation, weaken the immune system, harm cellular function, tend to discourage proper elimination, and are generally unhelpful for optimal hair growth.

Other substances to exhibit great care around when optimizing health and hair growth are coffee/caffeine (which is highly acidic and can leach nutrients), alcohol (recall the Nazarite vow excludes this, yet a glass of wine/single drink may be included occasionally if there is no addiction and no tendency toward addiction), cannabis, and any other psychoactive or consciousness-altering substances, including prescription drugs. These are best used with great discernement on a case-by-case basis - if at all - and if you are not yet seeing the results you want, it may be best to eliminate them for a time if you can. In general, the fewer addictive/intoxicating substances we can have in our lives, and the more amply we choose whole nourishment that is non-habit forming and non-altering of the nervous system, the easier it will be to regrow our hair - as we reattune our beings to nourishing frequencies instead of addictive/dissociative ones.

In addition, if you are in the process of replenishing a depleted supply of nutrients (which most of us are in need of), you may want to pay special attention to "anti-nutrients," especially phytic acid that can make absorption of nutrients difficult and even leach nutrients from the body. Phytic acid is found in most grains, nuts, legumes, and seeds in their unsprouted form and is a key reason that many people find grains difficult to digest. Fortunately, there is an easy solution to this, namely soaking and sprouting the needed foods into a much more bioavailable form that actually offers net-*positive* nutrients instead of net-negative ones.

Depending on how meticulous you want/need to be in order to absorb the needed nutrients and how much you rely on grains, nuts, legumes and seeds in your diet, this may be well worth implementing. The Weston A. Price Society offers a lot of free information on this topic and how you can implement it in your day-to-day food preparation (see for example: https://www.westonaprice.org/health-topics/vegetarianism-and-plant-foods/living-with-phytic-acid/). As I personally do not rely very heavily on grains, nuts and seeds, this is a moderate consideration in my diet, and I soak/sprout or simply purchase pre-soaked and sprouted grains, nuts, seeds and legumes as possible and as time allots. Experiment with what feels needed and best to you!

Light regular exercise will also help ensure good circulation to the scalp (gentle inversions such as those offered in yoga can be particularly helpful), while breaking a regular sweat helps to keep the lymphatic system flowing and support healthy detoxification and elimination, all of which matters for your hair.

Relatedly, there is also quite a bit to consider about eating and exercising correctly for your constitution and your own unique health and reproductive history (including family history). Because it's so individual, a full discussion of this goes somewhat beyond the scope of this book, but I will give a couple of examples of what I mean. Some people are constitutionally less grounded than others, carrying more "air" than "Earth"energies, and may need more grounding foods to stay balanced. People who are struggling with soul loss due to trauma and abuse may also find this to be the case, as I have. Such individuals may struggle with being vegan even though their spiritual friends tell them they "should," and may even become ill/weak if they do not consume enough highly grounding foods, such as bone broths and some meats. It is my fervent hope that people who are feeling less than optimal on a vegan protocol will consider eating some animal foods if/as beneficial, until such time as their energy configuration alters to allow new possibilities (which may or may not occur, but often does).

Alternatively, those with a slower, more grounded, "earthy" and/or "wet" constitution may thrive on a "high and dry" diet of primarily raw vegetables and well-selected grains, needing little to no meat at all, while becoming blocked and "weighed down" by meats and dairy. The surrounding culture of SAD might pressure the individual to pursue a diet of meats and another foods that can actually make a person of this constitution quite unwell - so once again, it is really up to the individual to "know thyself" and listen to their body, and theirs alone, in selecting the right inclusions and balance in their diet.

Proper hydration is also vital to healthy hair growth, and once again, varies between constitutions. One with a "wetter" and more generally grounded constitution may need far less water than someone with a "hot" or "airy" constitution. The best measure is that urine should be straw-colored, plentiful, and generally odorless. For the vast majority of us, waking up to a tall glass of fresh spring water (with a lemon wedge squeezed in, if tolerated) helps to start the day on the right footing regarding hydration and also helps to alkalize the body and support optimal cell health and growth.

In addition to eating and drinking according to personal constitution, it's vital to take full health history into account. For example, a woman who has just experienced a very heavy cycle or a miscarriage may experience strong cravings for red meat and/or organ meats to rebalance her system, whereas if that same woman - with identical constitution - had not experienced this, she may not have craved or desired those foods at all. Thus, it's important to take into context both basic constitution *and* personal history, and that these are complex and unique for every single person on Earth in ways that must not be minimized or leveled to "one size fits all" food dogmas.

If you are choosing to eat vegan while regrowing your hair, here are a few additional things to consider:

1) Be vigilant to get ample forms of protein and a full range of amino acids. Hemp seeds, chia seeds, buckwheat, quinoa, spirulina and pepitas are all considered "complete proteins," containing all needed amino acids and proteins; and can be enhanced/combined in your diet with many other protein-rich foods to be sure you are getting plenty.

2) Soaking and sprouting may be particularly important for you, because vegan diets may rely more heavily on grains, nuts, legumes and seeds (containing phytic acid) than diets that

include animal proteins. Note that most of the "complete proteins" listed above are grains and seeds, so these need to be soaked/sprouted for optimal nutritional value.

3) Consider additional supplements - for example with regards to key minerals such as zinc, copper, iron and selenium. You will want to be sure that you are either eating enough foods that contain these naturally, or supplementing in the correct ratios with supplements made of bioavailable food sources. I found this article helpful in providing information of plant-based foods that contain key nutrients: http://gentleworld.org/vegan-sources-of-vitamins-minerals/. If you are a menstruating woman, sufficient iron is particularly important and you may wish to supplement. Vitamin D is another key nutrient to attend to, both through supplementation and sufficient, safe sun exposure.

4) Use soy with caution. Although touted as a superfood for vegans and used in many vegan products, soy in its unfermented form contains a huge amount of phytic acid *and* can potentially disrupt hormone/endocrine balance. As currently ubiquitously found in processed, prepared foods in the US, it is over 90% genetically modified and heavily sprayed with pesticides. Soy *can* be used beneficially, I feel, but this would entail traditional fermentation of organically grown soy. Many Asian cultures have longstanding traditions and cuisines that utilize such properly prepared soy, and are a wonderful resource for those who wish to include soy in their diet. Our family has chosen to avoid soy altogether, and we suffer no ill effects due to its exclusion.

For those readers who would like to explore all of this complexity more fully, I offer services to dive more deeply into your constitution, health history and current needs, and custom-create a plan for optimal health that takes all into consideration.

As a start, the reader is invited to simply explore his or her ayurvedic *dosha* (constitution) by taking a short, free quiz online (for example: https://yogainternational.com/article/view/dosha-quiz); and of course strongly encouraged to follow your intuition and body's own wisdom and guidance at every turn.

To conclude this chapter, my general counsel regarding nutrition is to go (what feels like) *way overboard* in supplying yourself with amazing, healthy, fresh, nutrient-dense food. If you think you "need" one big plate of fresh greens, eat two or more. If you eat avocado here and there, eat it daily. If you drink organic smoothies once or twice a week, commit to having one daily with all the good stuff thrown in. If you are strict about refined sugar, be even stricter - but replace that with delicious, sweet fresh fruits and just a touch of real maple syrup or raw honey. There is no deprivation encouraged or necessary, as the abundance of living foods delights the palate and nourishes the body. See if you can make nearly every food that crosses your lips a superfood, with zero empty calories. Prioritize high quality, organic, well sourced food at the "expense" of buying more stuff that is simply stuff! Our family even radically downsized to a much smaller home in a less expensive area so that we could prioritize nutrition in the very highest for our family, and we are all greatly healthier for it. And this is the level of commitment generally required to have a truly positive impact on your health and hair.

Following is a sample menu of how I would optimally eat for a day in order to properly nourish my growing my hair:

Upon waking: Tall glass of spring water with lemon; cup of decaf coffee with raw cream.

Breakfast: Green smoothie with some combination of avocado, spinach, kale, other greens, beets, pineapple, blueberries, spirulina, and collagen, possibly chia seeds and cacao, one spoonful Camu Camu powder (vitamin C) pomegranate juice, apple juice.

Supplement with: One Viviscal tablet, one fish oil capsule, one black currant oil capsule.

Morning Snack: Paleo salmon bar by Epic or pastured, organic egg on sprouted toast.

Lunch: Big salad with romaine lettuce, greens, avocado, olives, chicken or shrimp, carrots, tomatoes, potatoes, feta cheese; dress with olive oil, apple cider vinegar and crushed garlic. Mug of homemade chicken bone broth.

Snack: Fruit salad of fresh berries with lemon and touch of honey, handful of pepitas

Dinner: Wild salmon with baby bok choy and sweet potato, doused in butter and hemp seeds. Second cup of bone broth.

Supplement with: One Viviscal tablet, one teaspoon Green Pastures fermented cod liver oil, one black currant oil capsule, one pomegranate extract.

Before bed: cup of locally sourced, raw milk.

I hope you will experiment with the information in this chapter, in your quest to develop the perfect style of eating for you: uniquely your own, deliciously nourishing, and bringing forth your inimitably beautiful shine from the inside out, which will soon result in even more luminously healthy hair! Now let us turn directly to the hair itself, and how to engage with and lovingly handle your hair as you navigate the healing process.

CHAPTER 4: *Hair as Sacred Antenna; the Proper Handling of Hair*

Before I outline the three stages of the Nazarite method, let us briefly discuss general handling of the hair so that you can use this information during all three phases of this protocol. You may need a few tools such as a wide-tooth comb and a natural bristle brush to keep your hair well cared for and styled according to your preference. But even more importantly, you may well end up discarding or gently placing to the side a whole host of other tools and products, such as blow dryers, curling irons, chemical dyes and harsh styling products, in your process of revealing the beautiful strong hair that has always been yours!

The truly wonderful news is, there is hardly anything needed by way of tools and products to nurture your hair into its optimal condition. While most (at least in the US) have been conditioned to seek a "holy grail" product as an end-all solution, I have found that hair products are far from the most important element of healthy hair and may well be the least. In my perspective, they should be treated as the "icing on the cake" of a rigorous, comprehensive protocol that addresses energetics, nutrition, full body/being care, and lastly, high quality topical products that will help and never harm your hair.

As for your actual physical touching/grooming of your hair, I recommend that you handle your hair as gently as you possibly can throughout this entire process, including and especially in the initial detox phase. To begin, please refrain whenever possible from touching or even looking at your scalp or hair out of frustration, self-loathing, despair, nitpicking criticism or worry. Please also refrain from gouging or scratching your scalp with your fingernails, as this can introduce bacteria. You may need to invest in becoming more conscious of your habits with regards to your hair, unpacking any layers of defeatism, shame or lack of self worth and replacing these with loving acts of self-adoration and peace.

In addition, you will want to be extremely mindful about who is allowed to touch and interact with your hair and in what manner, including your partner if you have one, your friends, family, hairstylists, etc. Anyone who wishes to interact with or touch your hair in any way should be coming from a place of love, not criticism or control, and should only introduce the most loving and nourishing touch to your hair. Choose your stylist wisely, and you may wish to keep your hair in your own gentle hands (literally) for a time until you feel confident that those touching your hair are loving and well intentioned. If - and only if - the connection is a loving and nourishing one, then by all means allow all adoration and affection to be bestowed upon your beautiful hair. :)

I also recommend that you place to the side as much of what can be damaging and stressful to your hair as possible, at least for phases one and two of this method (and by phase three, you probably won't even miss them!). This includes but is not necessarily limited to: chemical hair colors and dyes; chemical hair sprays, gels and styling products; curling irons, blowdryers; and straightening agents or perms. All you will need by way of products is a simple (organic or as close to it as possible) shampoo; a simple organic conditioner; and some basic organic oils - such as coconut, argan and marula - to style and control any frizz. My suggestions for all of these can be found in

36

Appendix C; and by all means please continue to explore to find the products that are best for you! Some people forego shampoo altogether, opting for no-pooing or co-washing. These options are discussed later in this text, and even more thoroughly in the book *Curly Girl: The Handbook* by Michele Bender and Lorraine Massey - and may be particularly good alternatives for those who, like me, have naturally wavy or curly hair.

You are also encouraged to forego any use of invasive, tight clips and bands in your hair. To the greatest extent possible, do not pull your hair back or up severely, do not put your hair in overly tight braids, and do not use elastic in your hair. If you need to put your hair up/back, elect to use cloth ties, preferably cotton, and bundle your hair only loosely. There will also come a point when it may feel intuitive to cover or veil your hair to further protect it as a sacred antenna, which we will discuss more in chapters to follow.

In all of this, you will start to become more and more aware of the energetic circuit that is your body and being, of which your hair is one important receiver, if not the most so. There are infinite ways that you can further explore what it means to be a living energetic circuit for yourself, in order to learn how to maintain your own energy field as resilent and strong, to not allow your circuit to be siphoned or misused, and to devote your antenna/circuit to those energetic dynamics of love and health that feel most honoring to yourself.

For example, in my own process with healing, it became apparent to me that I was (mis)using my energy with regards to the internet and spending too much time in "the ethers" as opposed to the grounded, physical world that included my body and all that surrounded me. This energy misuse had an addictive quality and it was challenging to divest from it. When I decided to go "offline" in order to reclaim my energy and forge a different pattern for myself, I was amazed at the amount of energy *de*stabilization that I first encountered. This is because my energy was (co)dependent on the dynamics of internet overuse, and not at all used to being "at home" in my body. I actually experienced a physical tremor and quite severe "detox" symptoms in the course of breaking this addiction (some level of which is generally to be expected in the detox of any and *all* addiction, whether to a literal "substance," another person, or a dissociative habit). To assist this detox process, I was guided to lie in child's pose, with my legs tucked under my belly and my head toward the floor, and then to connect my (energetically clean) hands to my hair.

In this simple act, I was able to begin literally completing my *own* energetic circuit as opposed to looking to something outside myself to fill and complete it. It took commitment and courage, and was actually quite intimidating - even frightening - to undergo this process because I had never been fully able to hold myself/my own energy before, but over time I did indeed learn how to function as complete, a commitment that is ever deepening and refining. Working with my hair in this manner was absolutely essential to learning how to quite literally complete myself - *and*, in turn, becoming energetically complete was absolutely key to healing and regrowing my hair.

As I was in the throes of this, and my system was quite literally reconfiguring itself in real time, I continued to have profound and distressing physical symptoms that made it extremely difficult to get any true rest or sleep. I actually became terrified that I had a major neurological disease such as multiple sclerosis or parkinson's, yet I knew from previous experience in healing that energetic transformations can create intense physical symptoms, so I continued to operate in trust that I indeed was on the correct path to healing and simply experiencing a dramatic healing crisis.

One night in the midst of all of this, I woke up at about 2AM in a cold sweat and it was as though my insides were burning with fever, while the exterior of my skin was cold and clammy. I felt as though I had some kind of foreign body lodged in my neck and back and I was shaking uncontrollably. I told Hanan that something felt very, very wrong; I literally felt near death.

On the spot, Hanan conducted healing journeywork to assess the root of these bizarre symptoms and discovered that according to his shamanic sight, I had a huge, metallic, yet somehow living "router" lodged into my back, neck and the back of my head (the very site where the primary hair loss was occurring). This router was directing all of my energy - my intrinsic life force - out of the back of my body through a circuit and then along a wire with a dangling end, a "live wire" which had since become obsolete yet was still leaking life force in a big way, creating a real hazard. This was the "wire" that *used* to be connected into whoever/whatever had been using me at the time, via the internet or whatever else I had allowed to distract me and keep me out of my own body. Because I had followed the cues of "unplugging" my attention and energy from the internet as well as all potentially toxic relationships and dynamics, and brought this energy "home" to myself, my life force was still pouring out but there was nothing and no one "plugged into" it, for probably the first time ever. And, my system - used to being falsely "completed" in this codependent manner - had no idea how to be complete unto itself.

All of this had been causing the tremendous energetic symptoms and chaos that was registering as physical symptomology. Hanan, with the help of a special guide who performs energetic "surgery" if you will, removed the "router" from my back and plugged my energy circuit back into myself. From that day forward, I was a markedly different person, with a new capacity to hold my own center, set boundaries, not allow myself to be used, and direct my energy in productive ways that kept me in my own center and being rather than having all my energy unconsciously and uncontrollably flying out of my system to supply unaligned people and dynamics, thereby constantly depleting me.

I relate this story here in this chapter, because all of this is deeply connected to the true function of hair. Our hair is the "wire" so to speak, that receives information as well as being a profound access point to our vital life force and energy. Until we have cleansed any unaligned energy dynamics that are harming us and reclaimed this powerful antenna for ourselves, it can be misused - thereby damaging not only our hair strength, luster and ability to grow, but also depleting and even endangering our entire beings.

I cannot overemphasize how real this process is, and how important and vastly relevant it is to almost every single human being alive today, regardless of whether they've experienced hair loss, but especially in those cases. Most of us - due to abandonment, trauma, underparenting, isolation from the Earth, and all the other ills of society - still have energetically underdeveloped systems that literally do not yet have the resilience to hold their own power in self-completion. The vital work of learning how to complete our own circuit, to generate a true energetic overflow of vitality, health and essentially, magic - is at the very core of what humans need to do to become sovereign and free. You will almost surely experience your own version of this "completion" process as you work your way through this method.

Other explorations on this theme - of working with your hair as an antenna and your body as an energy circuit - include wearing a hat while barefoot in nature, such that grounding energy comes in through your feet and is "held" in the body having the head/hair capped; practicing gentle inversions in which your head is placed directly upon the Earth, allowing not only increased circulation but a direct connection to the ground; placing your feet in butterfly position (a variation of "lotus" position in yoga) and then lowering your head toward your feet, to connect the energy circuit of yourself; and many more. These gentle physical acts of self-completion and/or forming a circuit with the Earth's sacred frequencies, all promote our energetic self-completion and ability to sustain health. All of this should be done with care and attention, never forcing, with ample space for conscious reflection as to the impact these practices are having on you and the way that your energy is flowing. If it feels beneficial, continue; and if not, keep exploring. Also note that there may be some discomfort and "healing crisis" symptomology if you are moving through any fear and resistance in this process, which is again, highly likely. Continue to go at your own pace, doing what works for you, and trust that all you are doing *is* having a beneficial impact. Over time, this will become more and more clear.

With further regards to interacting with one's hair and promoting health thereby, one of the greatest assets to our hair's healing and regrowth process is the hair's own, natural oil. We can gently work with this sacred natural oil by allowing it to accumulate and be utilized between washes. Thus, wash your hair as infrequently as you can so that the natural oils have a chance to do their task of sealing the hair cuticle, smoothing and strengthening the strands. I washed mine for once a week for the majority of my hair's healing process, which seems a good baseline for many people.

Gentle Hair Massage to Circulate Natural Oils

In the couple of days before you wash, when the oil starts to feel plentiful, you can utilize extremely *gentle* massage to help boost scalp circulation, add love to your hair, and coat your hair with this beneficial oil. To start, you will want to make sure that your hands are clean. By clean, I don't mean by scrubbing them with invasive or harsh "anti-bacterial" soaps or anything aggressive. The kind of cleanliness I am referring to is primarily energetic and only secondarily to do with things like bacteria and physical impurities.

First, you will want to put down (and optimally, *away*) any electronic and internet-connected gadgets, and either wash your hands well or optimally bathe with the intention of clearing this energy from your hands, hair and body before you begin to touch your hair. (This is generally true for contacting/touching your hair, as EMFs and invasive energies/frequencies are associated with electronics and the internet, and are rarely beneficial to hair growth. Since the hair is a very sensitive receiver, we want to intentionally cleanse our hands of these energies before interacting with the hair.)

Next, sit or lie down comfortably and begin slowly and gently massaging your scalp with your fingertips, being mindful not to use your nails. You will feel your fingertips, and possibly your fingers too depending on the style you use, become coated with the oil of your scalp. Continue massaging in circles with your fingertips, gently addressing every area of the scalp. The goal of this is not to apply any pressure or even to stimulate growth. It's simply to lovingly circulate the oil that is already on your scalp, allowing your fingertips to be coated. It should feel relaxing and wonderful.

Next, smooth the natural oils, using your fingertips, onto the hair as a whole. Work your way from the scalp out to the hair strands, slowly introducing the oil to the hair. If your fingertips begin to feel dry, you can go back to the scalp, re-coat your fingertips, and then continue at the point along the hair shaft where you left off. For long hair, you may need to keep going back, coating your fingertips and continuing a number of times. Complete this process by massaging the scalp once more and applying the oil via your fingertips to the very end. This will help to seal in your hair's health and strength. If you can do this for two consecutive days before washing your hair, it will do a great deal of good. At the least, spend some time with it the night before.

As a note, some people prefer to use a natural-bristle brush to circulate and coat their hair with the natural oils, which is also fine and will serve pretty much the same intention. As a curly girl and also someone who is highly tactile, I have found it much easier to use my own fingertips; but either way is fine. However, I don't encourage brushing your hair daily, and never aggressively, as it can easily cause breakage. Go very easily, applying minimal pressure, and brush only when you wish to circulate the oil to your hair.

Whether using your fingers or a brush, you can do this scalp/hair massage each week. Once you get to phase one, do this the night *before* the key protocol (which you will soon learn). This will in turn be followed by washing - again, preferably no more often than once a week.

Washing Your Hair

When I wash, I use an organic shampoo, gently suds the scalp and work through to the ends, rinse and then follow with an organic conditioner, mindful to use only my fingertips for this process with light pressure, and not the nails. At this point I either work through any tangles with my fingers *or* rarely, if needed, I use a wide tooth comb extremely gently to work through any remaining knots. This is the only time I use a comb, when there is "slip" from the conditioner, and I use it extremely carefully and minimally to resolve tangles if there are any. I then rinse the conditioner.

At least during phases 1 and 2, I recommend using a high quality spring water for this final rinse, unless your tap water is of really superior quality. This felt important to me in the critical phases of healing, becoming somewhat less so as my scalp and hair have healed, but still preferred by me even now that my hair is feeling healthier and stronger. (You may wish to warm the spring water gently in the bath or sink before you use it, so it's not shockingly cold!)

Following rinsing, I then gently towel "scrunch" the curls, applying a small amount of oil (marula is my current favorite) and allowing the hair to simply air dry. If your hair is straight or you want a smoother style, you may follow a different procedure of gentle combing with a wide tooth comb. The more gently you can conduct this entire procedure, and the more minimally invasive in terms of chemicals, products and styling tools, the better condition your hair will ultimately be.

Let us now turn to phase one of the Nazarite Method, with all our tools and knowledge in place.

CHAPTER 5: *PHASE ONE - Detoxification & Eliminating Infiltration*

"A woman who cuts her hair is about to change her life."

-Coco Chanel

In this first phase (which can last anywhere from about one to three months), we really get serious and focused about what is causing the hair loss and what is needed to change it. Whether it's physical illness, nutrient deficiencies, hormonal changes, a lack of self care, addictions and codependencies that have allowed the hair to become infiltrated, or some combination of the above, we begin by getting to the roots - literal and metaphorical. You can start implementing the nutrition element immediately, to begin creating new fertile foundation from which new hair will quite literally sprout. In addition to that, now would be a good time to take out a journal and write down any insights you have about potential causes or issues regarding hair growth, how you are feeling about your hair, and what you would like to have happen as a result of this process. You can also commit, right at the outset, to being kind, gentle and loving to yourself throughout this entire process, trusting that there *is* a way through *and* that you are already more than enough exactly as you are. It is very natural to feel emotional and concerned about your hair, as it's an extremely profound symbol in our culture that represents a great deal in terms of power - including much that is scarcely understood and rarely, if ever, articulated. Take a deep breath into your deepest knowing (or as many breaths as needed to *really* feel it): that you are rite on your path, exactly where you should be, and that everything is possible. Use this feeling of serenity and trust as a true north to which you return anytime you may feel stressed or in despair about your hair.

In addition, now would be the perfect time to explore the option of growing out any hair dye/color and transitioning to your natural color, if you have not already done so. While this is of course optional, it's my belief that it will truly be beneficial to restore the health to your hair. This transition to your natural color need not be depressing or daunting, but rather a sacred process of revelation and rebirth. Remember that if you have natural silver hair and/or are transitioning, and would like any additional support with this process, *The Silver Circle* on Facebook is designed for precisely that, and has over four thousand members who are either in the process of transitioning to silver hair, or "veterans" who've made the full transition, and all are there to support others in making it safe, sacred, and fun. This thriving group is connected to an inspiring movement of many women and men who have decided to embrace their natural silver hair and show the world the power of self-love and capacity to shine by simply being themselves. And if you elect to continue coloring your hair for now, that is ok too! Simply apply the principles and phases of the method nonetheless.

In recalling a bit more about my personal story with hair loss and regrowth, I can remember how intensely emotional this initial stage was, for me. As articulated, I had been dangerously "hacked" by predatory and malevolent energies that were playing/preying upon my childhood wounding due to sexual abuse, as a means of siphoning my energy. (My first book, *She is One*, details the nature of this initial abuse and how the resulting trauma set me up for being further exploited and harmed through what was essentially a common martyrdom dynamic: namely, a way to make me feel responsible for "healing" others to my own detriment, which proved to be a great vulnerability for me until it was finally healed within me.)

My hair was falling out in handfuls and a palpable bald spot had appeared, as documented in the first chapter. In addition, my scalp begin to itch immensely and I found myself gouging my nails into it involuntarily in my sleep. Self care had been thrown out the window in this, and my changing hormones at 40 were likely not helping matters. I was scared, ashamed, in despair, and desperate for this nightmare to stop.

At the time, I remember feeling a very strong urge to cut my hair, as it was continuing to thin and began to look very ragged and unhealthy. I had a strong sense that I had the opportunity to be rebirthed in a huge way, and that one important key to reclaiming my power - and resurrecting *myself* from what surely felt like a "death" process - was to heed this call to cut the hair quite short and in effect, start completely over. I consulted a hair expert who urged me not to cut my hair and cited this would be a mistake and counter-intuitive to my ultimate goal of growing my hair long.

But ultimately, I knew in my soul that it was necessary to take the drastic measure of cutting off the majority of the affected hair, to begin to create needed, healthy separation from this dynamic of infiltration and to free myself of continuing to carry around the corrupted dynamics associated with it. When I went to my trusted hairdresser asking for the big cut, she commented to me that it looked as though the entire bottom half of my hair had been chewed on by demons - which was indeed an accurate description of its appearance, as well as what had all but literally occurred!

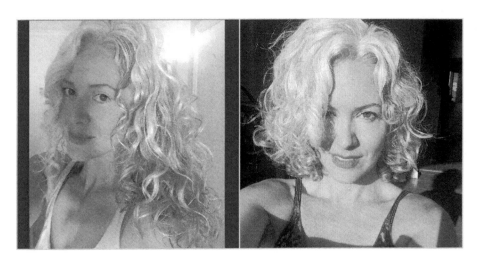

She cut my hair - as requested - into a chin-length bob (pictured above), which was the beginning of a healing process that would prove to be a long road requiring much more learning and commitment, but was a much needed start. Of course, it was not enough to simply cut the hair in order to sever the cords with this unaligned dynamic and the associated people; it was also imperative to trust myself enough to completely cut ties with the actual humans who were involved in this harvesting of my energy and to permanently change *myself* so that I was no longer compatible with this sort of infiltration.

At this juncture, I was still experiencing a lot of scalp itching and burning, and I knew there was more to do. My next step was to begin a detoxifying set of protocols with my hair, to gently cleanse the remaining hair of any impurities (both physical and in terms of energetic dynamics that were not serving), and to help gently relieve the hair follicles of any burdens in order to improve cell functioning, and to reset the microflora balance of my scalp and hair. I felt led to use an apple cider vinegar rinse for this; and was advised by a consultant to use it full strength on my head. I applied this to my hair and left on for just five minutes, shampooing subsequently. However, I found this to be much too strong and it left big red welts on my face and back where the vinegar had dripped down. I thus learned the hard way that some people are too sensitive to use apple cider vinegar at full strength, though it did seem useful as a natural detoxifying and cleansing agent. I waited a month after this, and was still itching! This time I applied a ratio of 2/3 apple cider vinegar to 1/3 spring water, and felt this balance much more gentle and aligned. It began to help.

At this time, Hanan's shamanic journeywork had also provided deep, really magical insights into a wonderful, key protocol that became the central practice of what we are calling the Nazarite Method. This simple, gentle, but incredibly effective protocol can be used in all three phases of this healing process to great effect, with minor variations to allow for which stage you are currently in. You can return to it again and again and use it as a focal point of your entire hair restoration process. A description of it is as follows:

Key Protocol of the Nazarite Method

1) In the bathtub or shower (bath is best), apply spring water to the entire head of hair, saturating every strand with the clear intention of washing/cleansing all unaligned dynamics, habits, attachments et cetera out of the hair. Visualize and feel this taking place as your hair is rinsed. State this intention (using this or your own carefully chosen variation/words): "I hereby ask and agree to release all dynamics, habits, attachments, and impurities (physical or otherwise) from my hair that do not serve the highest good at this time. I recognize the role they have played in my story and my growth, and I now release them, that I may embody the highest and truest version of myself as I am today." By using the expression "highest good," we elect to align our hair as an antenna/conduit of energy to that current energetic configuration and set of frequencies that are most beneficial for ourselves and all living beings at this time - recognizing that the full truth of this may be somewhat mysterious or unknown even to us, and allowing the intelligence of the energy that moves through us to guide us toward our own fullest potential, health and realization as our intention becomes realized.

2) Next, anoint your entire head of hair by pouring a well-chosen organic oil over your head (more discussion on which oil to use, when, to follow) - again taking care to coat every strand - with the intention of sealing *in* your own intrinsic life force, strength, truth, discernment, health and connection to source energy/nature/

creation. Visualize and feel this as so. You can state the following intention (using this or your own words): "I hereby seal in my own life force, such that I am in union and harmony with myself, in accordance with the highest good of this moment. I agree to be present to myself, to honor my hair and my entire being to the highest of my capacity. I take full responsibility for being able to hold my own power and to accept health, vitality and joy into my life, making any changes necessary to have this be so. Today, I honor and love myself."

3) Now allow this treatment to sit on the hair for a minimum of half an hour, and up to a full day (depending on what oil you are using, what phase you are in, and how much time you have, to be discussed in more detail below). Just a note that if you keep this on for a substantial length of time and choose to exit the bathtub, you will need to wear something you don't mind getting oily and/or put old towels down wherever you go!

4) Shampoo the oil out of your hair with a gentle, preferably organic shampoo. You may have to repeat this process to remove as much oil as you desire. Condition, rinse and gently style. Avoid harsh chemical or heat processes at this time, with natural air-dry being preferable.

Thus, to reiterate: the total weekly procedure including the key protocol will go in the following order: 1) lovingly massage to circulate your scalp's own natural oils and beneficially coat the hair (preferably the night or two before washing); 2) apply the key protocol with the stated intentions to purify and seal the hair; 3) wash and condition with organic products; 4) dry naturally with minimum styling products (preferably organic oil only). In a moment we will discuss the specifics for each phase, but this basic weekly procedure will remain constant throughout all three.

As an incredible "side" note that may be more central to those who are in romantic partnership, it was also shown to us that there is a wonderful opportunity for those in healthy, committed union to practice a really lovely form of intimacy and bond-building through this protocol. By asking one's partner to perform the loving acts of rinsing and "sealing" one's hair, the antenna of the hair receives and becomes connected and bonded to the other, through the love that transpires in this interaction. This very simple ceremony can be used to rekindle love between partners, to help people recover from the dynamics of sexual abuse and trauma and gently turn toward divine love, and more. Please note that this only works if you have a genuinely loving and supportive partner and is not advised if you are in anything that could be considered an "abusive" or codependent relationship! And, if you are not in a partnership and/or opt to perform this simple protocol on your own, it will still be equally powerful and effective.

The following chapter contains more information about this aspect of the protocol for those who are interested in exploring it more deeply. I encourage everyone to read it regardless of whether you have a partner that you wish to practice this with - ideally *before* beginning to practice the key protocol - as it contains potent and relevant information about sacred bathing and ritual that applies to everyone.

In the first stage of my own healing process (after I had already cut my hair quite dramatically), I created a detoxification blend of olive oil and garlic for the "sealing" aspect of the key protocol. This oil was specifically chosen by me for maximum, yet gentle purification of the scalp and hair, seeking to resolve the itchiness and inflammation while allowing my hair to "right" itself as an antenna of the sacred.

Garlic and Olive Oil Infusion (Detox & Nourish)

Simply place 6-8 peeled garlic cloves into a cup of olive oil (both organic), and heat gently on the stove for fifteen minutes or as long as desired. The oil should be on quite a low heat setting so that it does not bubble or boil, and the garlic should not turn very brown in this process (a tiny bit of browning may be inevitable). Allow the oil to cool to room temperature (or slightly warmer, to your preference), then place the oil in a glass container for your use in the key protocol.

The reason this particular oil combination is potent for detoxification is that the garlic is anti-bacterial, anti-fungal, anti-inflammatory, and contains a great number of nutrients such as sulfur, selenium, and B vitamins, all of which support hair growth. Olive oil, in turn, is deeply moisturizing and contains antioxidants, agents that inhibit any hormones that damage hair follicles, as well as components that stimulate new growth. Together, these two agents offer a great way to gently detox the scalp, reset microflora balance, cleanse excess hormones, and nourish the hair. This treatment can be left on the hair for a minimum of half and hour and a maximum of one hour, and then washed out with organic shampoo. (In the rare instance you feel any burning of the scalp after applying this, please shampoo out immediately, and then try again at a later date with a just three or four cloves infused in the same amount of oil, as this treatment should not burn or harm the scalp in any way.)

In the first few applications of the key protocol, my husband Hanan applied this mixture to my hair after the spring water rinse, as I stated the intentions as written above in both cases - thereby literally washing the old dynamics out of my hair in a powerful purification, while sealing in my own life force. We repeated this process once a week for about three weeks (after which we continued the key protocol weekly, but switched to olive oil alone).

This practice had an extremely potent effect on me. I could feel the old dynamics, addictive patterns, etc. losing their hold on me, while my own ability to stay grounded, present and true to myself increased with each round. My scalp stopped itching and I could feel that important transformation was under way. At this time, I chose not to look at the bald spot on the back of my head or wonder about growth, I simply continued to stay the course of washing the old dynamics out of my hair and sealing in the new, noticing what was arising with each round and taking positive action as it unfolded.

Also important - and highly related to this initial detox phase of the key protocol - is the topic of committing to regular digital detoxification. As discussed briefly above, I feel this practice is absolutely essential not only for optimal hair health but for living a vital, balanced life in an era when we are constantly bombarded with frequencies designed to infiltrate and even hijack our nervous systems - with our hair being a primary antenna and target of/for this infiltration unless we are careful to protect ourselves. These frequencies, and the dynamics which are encouraged and transmitted through/by them, can have the very deleterious consequence of fragmenting and fraying human consciousness and degrading our nervous systems (also as reflected in/connected to our hair), while we become addicted to and exploited by them - *if* we are continuously bathed in them with no awareness of how to shut them off and reset our nervous systems and energy fields to natural (Earth-based) frequencies, which are our biological "home" as organic beings and which truly nourish our nervous systems and total selves.

Thus, I found it of utmost importance to implement a weekly digital detox in accordance/synch with the key protocol outlined above, which in my case corresponds to the Jewish practice of *shabbat*, starting at sundown on Friday evening and spanning through sundown on Saturday (25 hours total). During this digital detox, I do my best to turn off as much EMF "noise" and as many artificial frequencies as possible, including turning off my router, my cell phone and even our electricity if I can for that time period, and purposefully return to a much simpler way of life. I light candles in the evening, spend quality and focused time with my family, go for walks and/or meditate in nature, and conduct the bathing and key protocol with as much time and presence as possible. This weekly, profound "reset" of the nervous and energy system cannot be overstated in its power and I truly feel that it's one of the keys to not only surviving, but thriving, in an era of chronic overstimulation and constant bombardment with EMFs.

I have found that all of this information that I discovered while in my own healing process can be implemented quite simply for others by using it as "map," while customizing it to the individual's own needs. In working with others, the very same principles and steps - with variations to suit the individual - nearly always apply. By now, you have likely already begun to adopt the nutrition and "hair handling" information given in the previous chapters. Now, you can also begin to implement the following, catered to your own needs:

Applying Phase One of the Nazarite Method

1) (Optional, but extremely helpful): Employ shamanic journeywork or other highly ethical and effective energy work, if possible, to kickstart the healing process, receiving energetic "diagnostic" information about the root cause of the hair loss and allowing the work to effectively push the "reset" button on your energy, breaking old patterns and making way for a profound rebirth to occur along with your new hair growth.

Regardless of whether the cause(s) are physical, emotional, energetic - or all of the above - this type of work, done well, will really help. We have found this work to be particularly important for men who are wishing to regrow their hair after long-term loss due to male-pattern balding, as the energy work can repair and reactivate long-dormant or damaged follicles in ways that little else can, giving these cells a chance to grow hair again. That said, it is truly divinely helpful for anyone and everyone seeking to regrow their hair. This work has been an unspeakably important asset in my own regrowth process and highly recommended to anyone.

As discussed above, my husband Hanan Eisenman is one such highly skilled and heart-centered shamanic practitioner and his work is really the "author" of the

Nazarite method in many ways. More information about his work can be found in the "resources" section at the end of this book, where I detail a special offer and discount given solely to readers. And if you elect not to do this step or it's not a fit for you at this time for whatever reason, the protocol will still help a great deal, so please read on!

2) Tune deeply into your own guidance/wisdom with regards to the level of detoxification that is necessary - if any - per the considerations that have been offered in this chapter. The details of this will be different depending on the cause and specifics of your own hair's history, needs and any hair loss you might be experiencing. At the very least, strongly consider implementing a weekly digital detox. Whether you are only able to allocate a few hours or a full day, this will make a marked difference in your energy. You can then allocate this time that you have set aside as special and sacred to begin utilizing the key protocol of washing/sealing your hair with focused intention, as described above.

In addition, if/as it's feeling necessary, one of three levels of detox specifically for the hair may be useful (listed from most to least intense):

★ (Most intense) Cut your hair significantly as a ceremony to release the old and begin the new. Retain the clippings and dedicate these either to the sky (by burning) or the Earth (by burying) signifying a completion of that chapter of your life, that will make space for your rebirth. This would be the most rigorous and "drastic" of the three options, yet when needed it can feel so wonderful to release whatever you need to let go of, and find a new sort freedom. Your intuition and knowing will tell you if this is needed for you and to what extent; you need merely tune in and listen. In no way should this feel like a rash decision or a "lashing out" or a masochism; it should feel good and empowering - otherwise please don't do it, or give it more time until it becomes clear. This is a big step, not undertaken lightly, and is not necessary or called for in all cases.

★ (Less intense) Use one or more applications of apple cider vinegar before beginning the protocol. As noted above, I used a ratio of 2/3 vinegar to 1/3 spring water to obtain the correct result for my sensitivity level. Leave on for no more than five minutes, and then shampoo out gently with organic shampoo. Continue with your regular hair routine. You can repeat this step up to two more times over the course of the next couple of months, but I don't recommend using the vinegar more than once a month or more than three times overall, in this phase. Again, this step is optional but recommended if you feel you've had a high level of infiltration and/or you are experiencing any itching, burning or discomfort of the scalp.

★ Use one or more applications of the garlic-infused olive oil as the initial "sealing" oil of the key protocol, for a minimum of two cycles and a maximum of one month (four cycles). This is recommended for everyone for at least the minimum, as it will help to reset the scalp and cleanse the follicles while simultaneously nourishing. Although a bit stinky (unless you, like me, adore and can't get enough of garlic!), this is a great and usually very helpful start.

3) Tune into your hair/body again and see if your hair feels different and the path to healing more direct and clear. While continuing to employ all the nutritional information, you can now ease off the garlic-infused olive oil if your scalp is feeling balanced, and prepare to proceed to phase two, which follows in Chapter 7.

CHAPTER 6: *Sacred Bathing & Optional Divine Union Considerations*

As articulated in the preceding chapters, sacred bathing and the key protocol of purifying/sealing my hair has been an extremely potent practice in my life. When I engage in this in the self-created sanctuary of the bath, I spend a good amount of time covered in the oil, completely devoted to allowing it to fully penetrate my hair and body, taking care to wash just as carefully and meticulously. It is a fully immersive (literally) ritual experience. This is very akin to the original ritual of baptism, practiced by the paleolithic Hebrews long before it was adapted by Christians - used to achieve and maintain energetic hygiene and clarity of the physical vessel, such that our life force is fully aligned and devoted. (We describe this ritual and other aspects of paleolithic Judaism in much more detail in our book, *God is with Us*, for anyone who may be interested.)

In this personal practice that I perform weekly, there is nothing more important and no place that I'd "rather be." There are no phones, no to-do lists, and no distractions. All of this gives rise to a deep sense of presence, magic and contentment that I honestly do not encounter nearly as often outside the bath. It has a sacred and ceremonial quality of purity and total peace and the "seal" of my energy is palpable, creating an energetic sanctuary of selfhood and completion in which I no longer feel any draw to anything that is unaligned or addictive, aka anything that would take me outside of myself.

Once we have cleansed all the oil and exited the sacred chambers of the bath, we may find that we are, in a very real sense, reborn. This is a wonderful time, once you emerge from the bath in this delicate rebirth, to *stay* in/with this new vibration for as long as you possibly can. You may find that the old things that "pulled" at you in an addictive fashion feel less appealing, while there is more spaciousness in your being for breath and the present moment. But in a strange way, it can actually be difficult to hold this vibration even though (or possibly *because*) it feels so much cleaner and healthier. You might feel the tug of the rote behavior, the desire to "busy" yourself again or otherwise indulge in a distracted habit. See if you can stretch yourself to stay "in" the purified, expanded vibration just a bit longer each time, holding that "seal" as you build your own personal power and ability to be in simple presence and completion.

If you are in the process of healing your hair and are currently in a loving, committed partnership, here are some extra recommendations and ways you can use the Nazarite method to not only help regrow and strengthen your hair, but also to forge a beautiful, healthy bond between you and your partner that is based in true intimacy and divine love. Let me emphasize again that - because hair is so sensitive as an antenna and our intention is to heal - I do not necessarily recommend these additions if your partnership is uncommitted and/or feels unstable or unhealthy in any way, and I also leave it to the reader to discern your own level of comfort and energetic safety with regards to this.

If you are undertaking the key protocol with a partner and are able to devote a full day, you can ask your partner to wash and seal your hair with the oil, and also to say the words of intention on your behalf as a "blessing," if this feels aligned. You can also allot time for each partner to have this experience one after the next, so that you ultimately get to experience this divine state of wholeness, presence and completion at the same time. I recommend doing this in a way so that each person gets their "solo" time in the bath and then the other can wash/anoint them as they are ready, also allowing ample space for alone time and self-reflection (as I have found that an important key is to not be too "on top" of each other, and to allow this state of being to arise organically). If that is not possible due to time constraints, you can "take turns" on alternating days in being the "anointer" and the "anointed" so to speak. You can experiment with it until it feels rite, and get into your own rhythm with this as sacred partners.

If you are in trusted and committed patnership, the time following the hair/bathing protocol can present a wonderful opportunity to explore divine intimacy within the energetic "seal" that you have created together. Whether this is sexual union or time spent vulnerably in intimate touch together, or both, this is a way to safely build the bond within the context of the sealed energy that you have created.

One simple ritual that I like, in this regard, is to anoint my husband's feet with my sealed hair, following his ritual of intention-setting and pouring oil over it. I conduct this once my hair has been rinsed of the oil, but while the energetic "seal" is still unbroken. By "unbroken," I mean specifically that I have not "returned" to or revisited any old habits, dynamics or paradigms that do not "live" within the seal (only you will know what these are for yourself), but rather have kept my energy/hair sanctified and set apart for the present/union. I then kneel on my knees and bless my husband's feet with my hair and say words of thanks and adoration to him, in gratitude and love and acknowledgement of his aligned masculinity and total being.

Because of the energetic nature of hair, this has the effect of completing the cycle that began with him pouring spring water on my hair to "cleanse" and bless it. Just as he has lovingly blessed my hair, so I bless his being with my hair, and this creates a living, loving divine union circuit between the two. If you are in a loving partnership and decide to implement this, you may well be absolutely astounded at how this simple set of rituals deepens and transforms the love between you.

If you are *not* in a partnership of this nature, you can still use this time when your energy is "sealed" potently by conducting any further intention setting or ceremonial work that you feel called to at this time. Because your energy has been "trued" and brought "home" to you through the sacred bathing, anything you choose to direct your energy toward at this time will be greatly magnified compared to when you are distracted or enmeshed with any unaligned frequencies even slightly. Thus, if you have any form of "manifestation" or aligned sacred ritual work that you already practice, this would be a wonderful time to direct your full focus toward that and see increased capacity to realize your goals and dreams. With or without a partner, the time following the key protocol when your hair and energy are still "sealed" will likely be a potent time to work with your own life force, call in that which is sacred, and notice that which is shifting. With all of this in mind and heart, let us continue to the second phase of the method.

CHAPTER 7: *PHASE TWO - Nurturance and Active Regrowth Protocols*

"Caring for hair is very important, for like the Sweet Grasses of our Mother, the Earth, our hair holds the purity of our intent. For our thought can purify the thoughts of others. Native children are taught to wash and rinse hair, and are taught the proper use of the gifts of the Plant People; learning which bulbs, roots and herbs, will bring luster and light to one's hair. Maintaining the health of one's hair is important, as is maintaining all physical and spiritual health and wholeness."

-Paula Lightening Woman Johnstone

At this juncture of your healing process following its detoxification and given your new commitments to the key protocol, your hair can ritely be thought of as a newborn baby, being freshly introduced to what is possible. You have released a good deal of the patterns and dynamics that were inhibiting hair growth and/or causing harm, while nurturing yourself with excellent nutrition and nourishing hair oils, and have re-dedicated your energy - via your hair - to your own highest good and well being through the purification and "sealing" protocol outlined in the previous chapter. You may have chosen to cut your hair, or simply to have detoxed through the apple cider vinegar and garlic-infused olive oil treatment, but regardless of how intense this process needed to be in your particular case - a real transformation has taken place and something new has been born.

Thus, the way that as you would protect and treat your very own newborn baby is exactly how you will ideally view and care for your hair at this juncture. When a baby is first born, we keep them especially close and nurture them extra much. They are affectionately swaddled and cuddled, encouraged to sleep often, eat the softest, most digestible food in the world, and nothing is expected of them except to rest and grow as they slowly change and develop. All of this applies quite literally to your hair at this stage.

To reflect on my own process for a moment, I remember being in this stage and what I was led to do to nourish my hair. Since, in my case, the hair loss was caused primarily by energetic infiltration, I felt especially protective of my hair and felt the intution to "swaddle" it (again like a baby) to, in effect, shield it from any unwanted energies having access to it/me. Since a significant part of the issue was my *own* (co)dependency or allowances of these energies that were in turn destructive, this was as much to keep unaligned energies "out" of my hair as it was to seal my own energy "in," to allow time and safe space for a new dynamic to form. This is true in nearly all - if not all - cases of codependency and addiction. It is our own "dependence" on destructive energies and dynamics that allows them to stay present in our lives and holds them there, so by placing a literal barrier between ourselves and them (or even more accurately between the old version of ourselves that would allow this and the *new* version which sets a healthier boundary), we disallow this dynamic from continuously prodding at - and threatening to re-open - a wound that is now seeking to heal thanks to the detoxification process we've already undergone.

This is what the process of veiling my hair was all about for me. For about a four to six month period in 2017, I chose to veil my hair and I honestly wasn't sure if this would become a permanent choice for me, or a temporary one. I was simply radically willing to change my entire relationship with my hair, to protect it as much as necessary for as long as I felt called to complete this transformation, and see what would happen.

In this process I discovered that another really important aspect of veiling is to actually witness and release the control mechanisms that are actually placed on our hair via society's demands. Particularly as women we are socialized to "perform" our beauty as a form of social currency that is pleasing to others and will maybe get us things like validation and success; our appearance is even often wrapped up with our core worth and sense of safety in terrifying ways. This of course applies deeply to our hair and the constant demands that many of us place upon it, often unconsciously. This issue affects almost all of us - certainly the vast majority of women, but men are also not immune to this dynamic. This above all is the deep reason why so many of us have been addicted to our hair dye, horrified to let our silver hair show as it would be some marker of "aging" or "letting oneself go" according to society's narrow judgments, and also the reason that so many of our torture our hair with untold curling irons and aggressive hair sprays etc., to try and get it to "perform" according to our own interpolated standards of what society wants and expects of us, or deems "beautiful." The stress of this alone can be a factor in hair loss and is well worth exploring on our path to healing and energetic sovereignty (which in turn, also helps us to grow healthy, beautiful hair).

As my online/public persona is somewhat symbolized/ recognized by my hair (particularly since I have grown out my natural silver), this was an opportunity for me in particular to take stock of the ways that I was allowing my hair to be "used" as a bartering chip of self-worth, identity, attention and validation and break any addictive dynamics that were going on with regards to this. I feel this is a healthy process for almost everyone - since one of the main reasons we place these demands upon our hair and ourselves is to meet with society's approval, and not necessarily intrinsic to ourselves or in alignment with our own highest good. Who are we when our hair is not focused on as a key part of our identity or associated with our worth? How does our hair look and feel when we are not asking it to perform? All of these were important questions to me when I decided to undertake the process of protective veiling.

Lastly, I wanted to veil my hair to give myself a break *from* myself, if that makes sense. Since I had lost a lot of hair and had a noticeable bald spot, I had a tendency to fixate on that spot and continuously, somewhat obsessively ask: *Was it getting better? Did it really look as bad as I thought it did? Would it be there forever?* I realized that this intense nit-picking and constantly inquisitive energy was not going to be helpful to my healing process whatsoever; it was just going to keep me in a loop of panic and low self-worth that would be counterproductive to healing. Thus, my decision to veil was also related to my own desire to accept myself exactly as I was in that moment and simply allow aligned growth and transformation to happen. Once I decided I was still worthy and (self-)loveable whether or not my hair ever grew back, it took the pressure off the healing process and actually allowed the amazing nutrition and the protocol the necessary time and opportunity to do its work, unimpeded by my overactive monkey mind.

I was also determined to have a lot of fun with this process (because life is short and all of this should be fun!), and to adopt veiling styles, hoods, etc. that felt compelling and beautiful to me and my newly emerging version of self. I started to play with cotton wraps, choosing a simple white cotton, and ordered a few styles of these (mostly from etsy), which felt light, breathable, loving and protective but *not* oppressive. I wore them during the day, with my hair loose at night. The only people who saw really me unveiled during that time were my husband and children and perhaps a couple of friends who are in my closest, most intimate circle and completely trusted by me.

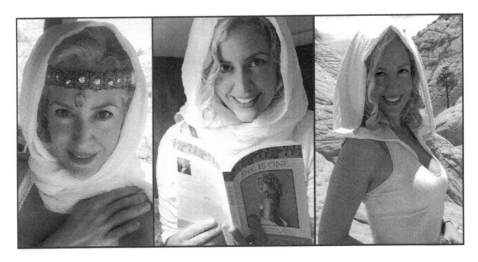

Above: a few images from my "veiling" phase in which I gave my hair the time, space and protection needed for full healing.

It's important to note that this decision did not feel like a "should" or "must" to me, as much of religious veiling would seem to. There was no external authority or organization telling me I "had" to do this, it was quite simply my choice. We could write an entire book on the fascinating topic of women's hair and why so many religions have dictated its veiling/covering -

with all of the power struggles and apparent patriarchical shaming and complexity that goes along with that topic - but suffice it to say simply that in my own situation, it was not under any form of coercion or external demand whatsoever that I chose to veil; nor did I see my hair as, in any way whatsoever, "bad," "shameful," "sinful," "provocative" (of sexual desire), or any of these notions that may seem connotated to women's hair in instances of religious veiling.

Parenthetically, I also have a deep sense that original veiling for women started during the matriarchy thousands of years ago (before the rise of patriarchal religion) amongst the priestess class, and had much more to do with the dynamics I am referring to here (protection, devoting one's antenna, cultivating divine power, and sacred vitality), than to do with anything shame- or control-based, which I feel came later when certan religions or religous sects co-opted earlier practices. So in a way, I was - in this process - recovering and reclaiming an (ab)original stance and purpose for the veiling of my hair as a woman. I was quite aware of this at the time and found it all extremely fascinating and powerful. And while the "charge" around men's hair is somewhat different - in that (appearance of) hair does not seem to be nearly as huge a part of identity, power struggles, and societal expectations for men as for women - I feel that all of these principles would and do apply generally to men, as well.

At the same time that I undertook the protective veiling, I was continuing the weekly massage to circulate and coat my hair with natural oils, the key protocol, and the organic shampoo/ conditioning routine, all as outlined in the previous chapter. In this phase, I opted simply for organic olive oil for use in the key protocol. Over time, this did cause my silver hair to yellow somewhat, but since I was veiling at the time, I did not mind. I decided to stick with this oil for a bit longer to see what its effects might be for me. (Since then, I have created a special set of recommendations for silver haired participants in this method, which I will detail later.)

I carried on like this for a period of perhaps three or four months, all the while not viewing the "problem" areas of my hair or really even looking in a mirror much at all (as it happens we were actually living in the wilderness with only one tiny bathroom mirror, so I found that I forgot to look at myself altogether for days or even weeks!). Funnily, I still felt a bit fatalistic about my hair and its recovery, as some glum part of me seemed still convinced it would not regrow (which was particularly ironic given that I have been witness to/recipient of so many physical miracles and know well the regenerative capacity of the body!). But one thing that I did know for sure was that my entire body was beginning to feel stronger, more solid, more resilient, more energetic. Just overall *better*. The evidence of hair loss (in the form of giant globs of hair in the drain) had slowed markedly, so I was hopeful I was going in the right direction. Hanan, my husband who had supported me throughout this process with his shamanic/healing work and administering of the key protocol, lovingly confirmed that I was indeed very much on the right track and continued to offer energetic support. I had also made enormous progress - via the weekly protocol - in purifying my being (via my hair) of unaligned dynamics of codependency, martyrdom, self-sacrifice, etc. so that my body and being were now functioning as a much more capable, functional healthy energetic circuit.

So, after these months of veiling and abstaining from even looking at my hair, one day I decided to take a peek at the back of my head where the bald spot was, and lo and behold it was gone! In its place was a solid tuft of hair sticking out of the back of my head, a clear regrowth in the exact site of the loss. Overall, my hair had grown thicker and stronger.

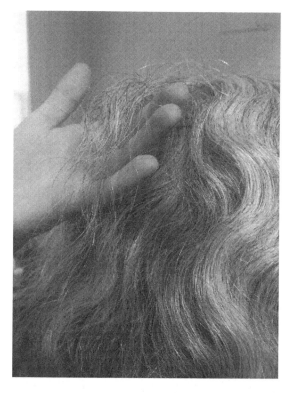

Above: my then nine-year-old daughter gently holding the "tuft" of regrowth in my bald area. I was so excited to see this months after I began the Nazarite method of reclaiming my energy and regrowing my hair, and after I had been veiling for some time.

At this time, Hanan journeyed again and he received some additional protocol information that would help us to expand the nurturing qualities of the key protocol, including some helpful new "ingredients." I introduced these additional healing agents (which I will detail in a moment) at this point, really once I was already seeing this great regrowth happening and knowing that I was truly on my healing path. However, I feel they can also be used as early as the beginning of the second

71

phase if one feels called, as they surely will not hurt and will likely only benefit the hair.

Applying Phase Two of the Nazarite Method:

To apply all the principles I've just articulated to your own hair, begin by asking yourself if veiling/covering or otherwise shielding/protecting your hair feels right for you, and to what degree. Only you know the answer to this. Perhaps you will choose to veil for only a short time, or for certain days of the week. Perhaps you will find another method of protection that feels helpful to you, such as tucking your hair safely in a braid or a bun (loosely, please)! Or perhaps this practice does not feel important or necessary for you at all. Take some time to truly tune into your own wisdom and heed what you receive, for yourself.

Whatever you decide with regards to veiling/covering, you can definitely choose to amp up the topical nutrient level of the key protocol at this time, while continuing to nourish yourself with increasingly amazing nutrition so your hair and entire self will shine from the inside out.

The additional agents that I was guided to use in my hair for the key protocol, to superpower its growth, are: pomegranate oil, raw (organic, pastured) egg whites, and aloe. Using these super nourishing beauty agents in addition to a carrier oil (you can either continue with olive oil or switch to coconut oil at this time) will add a new dimension of effectiveness to your weekly protocol and really produce growth and shine. Here is the why and how to use each:

- *pomegranate oil*: This oil has incredible healing properties for skin and hair, and has been considered a sacred oil since ancient times. It is amazingly hydrating, stimulates circulation to the scalp, strengthens follicles and will help grow stronger, healthier hair. Simply add 1 tablespoon of organic pomegranate oil per cup of carrier oil you are already using (I like either olive or coconut oil).

- *egg whites*: Using organic egg white on your hair is like a "protein pack" that gives your hair a chance to literally rebuild itself from the protein and other beneficial nutrients. I have found it can be a bit drying on its own, but added to the other ingredients of this "recipe" it adds many helpful building blocks that your hair can use. Add one egg white per cup of carrier oil.

- *fresh, organic aloe vera*: Aloe is one of the most benefical ingredients, bar none, that you can ever use on your hair. Aloe heals and stimulates damaged follicles, helps prevent further hair loss, stimulates hair (re)growth, nourishes hair with a variety of nutrients, and helps restore pH balance to the hair. To use in this protocol, it is best to procure a fresh organic aloe leaf. Fillet the leaf by removing the tough exterior "skin," then squeeze the slippery gel out of the leaf and put in your mixture. You really don't need much, perhaps a tablespoon of the gel will do. This leaf will usually save in the refrigerator for at least one additional week, so you can reuse it again a second time. If you cannot find a fresh leaf, you can use a bottled aloe gel, just make sure that it's organic and as close to nature (with as few additives) as possible.

With all of these ingredients, there is room to experiment with quantity and even decision to include, or not, in your key protocol. Everyone's hair is different and will respond uniquely. I found that my hair looks the very best when I just use the oils -

while the other two ingredients, while nourishing, can actually feel drying if used too frequently. Thus, what I opted to do is to use the two oils combined for three of the four weekly uses per month, while saving the "full shebang" of all four ingredients mixed together for one special, monthly treatment. This is also more time-effective since filleting the aloe, etc. is a bit messy and time consuming. However, I would say that at least once a month it's worth going all-out to give your hair the full four-ingredient treatment, and don't forget to do the intention setting with both the initial rinse with spring water *and* the sealing of the hair with the treatment. In the case of using all four ingredients, you will want to wash the treatment out after just half an hour, as the egg whites can become hardened on your hair. Also rinse in warm but not hot, water; so your hair doesn't turn into an omelette. :) Be sure to play with the quantities of each ingredient and the frequency of the full four-ingredient treatment to see which way is best for you.

When I began to employ this more robust treatment to my hair during the key protocol, I saw even more gains to my hair, as it continued to fill in, grow at an increased rate, and look shinier and more resilent than ever. My hair grew rapidly and began to approach the length it was when I initially had to cut it in 2016, which was so fulfilling! It was at this juncture that I felt called to take an official Nazarite oath with regards to my hair, which you will read more about in the next chapter. Whatever you have decided with regards to veiling and the enhanced ingredients for the key protocol, you will also likely see huge gains in your hair growth and overall health too!

A FEW SPECIAL CONSIDERATIONS REGARDING SILVER HAIR

If you, like me, have a lot of silver or white hair (or have opted to begin transitioning your hair to its natural silver as a result of this protocol, which is wonderful), there are just a few things you may want to keep in mind. As mentioned above, olive oil can be yellowing over time if used as the oil for the key protocol. If this is a concern for you, you can try switching the olive oil for coconut oil at any time. I do recommend using the olive oil for the first phase (infused with garlic), during the detoxification process. But following this, it is okay to switch and you will likely see very similar benefits. As your hair moves into the second and third phases and *if* (and only if) you are beginning to see recovery/regrowth, I also think it's fine to use a well-sourced violet/purple color correcting shampoo minimally to maintain the silver color of your hair. Silver is special in that it can easily pick up and show any form of color deposit from our water, pollutants, etc. and requires a little extra maintenance in this way. Note that not all purple/toning shampoos are creasted equal and most tend to be very drying, which is far from ideal. I personally use the Aveda brand "blue malva" shampoo as needed (no more than once a week and usually more like once a month) to help keep my silver on track. They also make a conditioner of the same line, which I've found a bit more aggressively chemical, but can be used *sparingly* with the shampoo to also help correct color (I use it maybe once every three months). If you are not yet seeing regrowth and are still in the early stages of this protocol, I recommend avoiding the

Aveda for now and staying with the very gentle organic shampoos listed in Appendix C until you are ready. Per the stance of the early phases of this protocol, see if you can simply be okay with releasing aesthetic expectations and demands placed upon your hair while it's going through this intense healing and rebirth process. This grace given in the short term will likely pay off in a big way, in time.

CHAPTER 8: *PHASE THREE - The Oath, Maintainence & Further Dedication*

Heading into what we will call phase three - the final phase - of this protocol, I began feeling really good. I was amazed by the sheer depth of this process and how much it taught me and led me through, in my quest to better care for my hair and myself. By this phase, you too will likely be feeling really great about the transformation that has taken place, and starting to see notable favorable changes in your hair. Please remember that, for me, this phase started about six month in to the total process, so it did not by any means happen overnight!

If you are reading this book and have not yet fully implemented the first two phases, please do not become frustrated or impatient if you have not yet seen results. Remember that what you do to take care of your hair today will only become visible, on the deepest level, weeks or months from now. Take the time to go through the phases fully, remembering that this timeline is your own and will be different for every single person experiencing this.

At the very least, you will likely be experiencing noticeable signs that you are on the right track: an increase in energy levels, a sense of increasing peace with regards to your hair, a clarity in the self with regards to one's own energy use, as affects your hair. If you have gone through the first two phases organically and thoroughly and are not yet seeing the gains and breakthroughs you had hoped for, now is a good time to go back through this book and refine: Are you doing all that you can, nutritionally, to fortify your entire body and (re)grow your hair? Have you undertaken any form of energy work to help clear your own energy and diagnose the energetic roots of the hair loss or other obstacles to hair growth? Have you surrendered enough of the harsh and toxic products and heat-related tools that can stress hair out? Are you being extremely gentle and nourishing to your hair, as you would to a newborn baby, allowing it to be its own and not made to "perform" for society? Are you being mindful of your personal boundaries and who has access to your being/hair?

Take a moment to feel into these questions, and if you find there is more work to do, dig more deeply and commit to this new level. Remember there is no judgment in this whatsoever, it's purely the process of learning to nurture and nourish yourself, and everyone's conclusions and results will vary. Remember you can also take breaks from all of this if it begins to feel unproductive or frustrating, and simply return at any time that feels right to you.

You may also, at any time, feel the need to cycle back through phases one and two even if things are going nearly "perfectly," just as a matter of maintenance. For example, well into phase three I started experiencing some scalp itching again after a hot summer and a family cross-country move, so I elected to return to phase one and conduct an apple cider vinegar rinse, then nourish my hair with a week of covering, as in phase two. This brief cycle through the earlier phases serves to deepen the gains, and it's great to know that you can return to an earlier phase anytime that it feels aligned to do so, for as long as you want or need.

If you are at this stage, like me, feeling great about the progress you have made, and more devoted to growing your hair than ever, then you may wish to consider taking an oath to dedicate your hair as a permanent conduit only of the highest and most aligned energies for yourself. Although it has its origins in the Nazarite oath described in Chapter 1, this oath needn't be religious in nature but rather intentional and energetic. It is, however, still energetically binding and not something to be taken lightly (as with any vow). That is why I encourage you to consider this at the "culmination" of your work with this method, rather than at its inception. It is something whose commitment we grow into, as much as it continues to grow in us.

When you vow your hair in this way (I am here using vow and oath as interchangeable), you are vowing the primary antenna/conduit of energy of your entire being to the highest and most aligned course of action for yourself. You are essentially saying that you've agreed to leave behind certain aspects of current "social norms" - such as relying on your hair as a bargaining chip of any form of approval, or letting your hair be infiltrated or used in any way - while allowing your hair to be *itself*, dedicated to its own sovereignty. By extention, this sovereignty becomes true in a sense for your total self through the undertaking of this oath. This is no small matter and its power should not be understimated.

At the point in which I felt ready to take this oath for myself, my hair was just about to cross the threshold length at which I had cut it in 2016. After I took it, it rapidly flew across the threshold and is now far longer, and far healthier, than it has ever been in my entire life, with no plans to stop growing it. What I have pledged is that 1) my hair - and by extension the entire energy circuit that comprises my being - is dedicated to the highest good and none other; 2) I will grow my hair for at least a year at a time with no trims or cuts (with option to rededicate and renew the vow following any trim); 3) When I do choose to trim, I will devote the trimmed locks to the sky or Earth (as previously discussed).

Applying Phase Three of the Nazarite Method - The Oath

If you feel ready and wish to take this oath for yourself, you will simply go to a field, a sandy beach or other place in nature, and draw a circle on the ground. You will stand in the center of the circle, and recite the following words: "I hereby pledge to complete myself and become a vessel of the sacred, whole and sanctified. I pledge my hair to the highest good, for the duration of this oath." You will then pour fresh water on the circumference (circle's perimeter) for the full 360 degrees, making sure to complete the circle to seal in and affirm the words you have spoken. At this time, after a few deep breaths into this intention, you may exit the circle as you choose. Returning to this site as feels helpful will be an empowering way to remember the commitment that you have undertaken.

While it would seem perhaps odd (to some) to say that this simple oath could have any potential impact on hair growth and health, I have found that making this commitment for myself has greatly magnified my overall health and vitality, as well as offering a transcendent feeling of joy and beauty to my life that I can really only describe as miraculous. Many - if not all - of us stuggle with being continuously and fully embodied in a time when distractions and manipulations abound. The simple words "I pledge to complete to myself," mean that we agree and commit to staying in our own center and sovereignty, uniting our energetic essence with our bodies. And in citing the second line, "I pledge my hair to the highest good," we are agreeing to dedicate our hair and ourselves to the highest good not merely in the once-a-week key protocol, but continuously, for all of time. Again, this commitment is real, with actual energetic consequences, and not to be undertaken without true readiness - but if you do feel ready for this step it is both a wonderful culmination *and* a potent accelerant to this process.

Consider transitioning to "no 'poo" method

Additionally, you may find your relationship with the key protocol of the Nazarite method (the weekly intention setting and washing/sealing) evolves, as through the weekly cleansing and devotional practice, you become more and more able to hold the vibration of clarity and focus in your energy field - and specifically the sacred antennae of your hair - with regards to what energy/dynamics you are and aren't transacting. For example, after some months it felt to me personally that the "cleansing" process became less and less necessary in order to wash unaligned dynamics, additions and habits out of my hair and being and seal in the aligned ones, as I became able to hold and maintain the sacred, aligned frequencies and energetics for longer and longer periods of time of my own accord and due to a sort of sacred momentum cultivated by this practice.

At the same time, my scalp began to feel different overall, less itchy and with less urge or feeling that it needed to be washed. I began to space out the time between washing and sealing, going a month or more without needing to apply any shampoo to my hair, and simply either rinsing as needed with spring water to reset the style and appearance of the hair and gently cleanse the scalp; or "co-washing" (minimally cleansing with a gentle, organic conditioner only) to reset the style and look of my hair as needed.

At the time of this writing, I have felt content and nourished in conducting the key protocol of washing/sealing with intention just once a month and using either no-pooing or co-washing inbetween. One of the great benefits of this practice is that we get to keep our hair's own beneficial oils for much longer, which helps to seal the cuticle of the hair and keep it strong so it can grow longer and remain in great condition. However, if at any time I feel "gummed up" or "weighed down" by what my hair is carrying; or "addicted" to anything outside myself by way of attachments that have found their way into my system via the hair antenna, I simply return to the weekly protocol with renewed intentions until I'm feeling back on track. A once-daily bath in simple water, with or without rinsing my hair, is generally enough to keep my energy on track. All in all, it's a continual work in progress, a dance with my own energy and mindful witnessing of where my energy is going, what I'm receiving (i.e., what has access to my energy field), and whether I'm able to stay in my center in a true "overflow" state. All of this takes practice!

In addition, I have been guided to ease up on some of the meat and animal foods while increasing salads and vegetable/fruit based smoothies, and keeping well-sourced fish and some seafood as a primary means of certain nutrients as detailed earlier. Similarly, your needs will likely shift throughout this process, and that is why listening to one's own body and knowing is so absolutely essential.

If you continue this process for some time with focus and devotion, you may well find, as I have, that although the clock is ticking and you are (according to society's narrow view) supposed to be 'in decline,' you are in fact feeling younger and younger, more and more vibrant, more and more alive and capable, and more and more true to yourself. You may discover that the entire concept of growing older as some kind of 'loss' is truly a manufactured farce to keep us falsely worried, self-loathing and impoverished - while truly we become richer in wisdom and fortitude, more beautiful and more vital with time. What began as a quest to grow longer, stronger hair may have radiated out and become a total-life, total-self transformation for the better, one that just keeps on expanding and emanating in ways you never could have seen coming. This is certainly true in my case; and I will share a bit more about my personal transformation in the concluding chapter to follow. Whether or not you have decided to culminate your journey with the Nazarite method with the formal oath (a culmination which is always truly just a new beginning), I congratulate and honor you for the amazing work that you have put in - in this process - on behalf of yourself, your body, your hair, and really the whole world which benefits from *you* loving yourself.

CHAPTER 9: *CONCLUSION*

Thank you so much to everyone who has read and implemented the wisdom in this book. I hope you are seeing wonderful results and have perhaps also learned to regard your hair in a totally new way, as a profound conduit of power, and a symbol of your own inner beauty and devotion. Regardless of where you are in this journey in terms of results, I hope it has led to deeper self-honoring and acceptance from the deepest inside out, as our exterior radiates as a reflection of our deepest interior alignment. I hope you have also gleaned that the content of this book is multi-applicable, ever deepening and can be revisited with totally new and emergent results any time it feels compelling to you; the learning process is not only ongoing, but infinite. I'm looking foward to hearing feedback from many of you as to how this method is working for you, and continuing to support you on your journey of long, strong, beautiful hair!

As of this writing, my hair is the longest and best it's ever been. In full disclosure, I am still in process and *still* seeing new regrowth in the areas where I lost marked amounts of hair during my "lowest" point in 2016. Just in the past few months (already more than a year into this process), I've seen regrowth in my temple areas as I continue to refine and deepen the work with my hair and health, showing that this work does not happen overnight - but surely shows incredible rewards with dedication.

"Coincidentally" (I think not), as my hair continues to regenerate I am also feeling the best and most vibrant I've ever felt in my entire life, bar none! I have completed a great deal of healing of deep trauma, have learned to set healthy boundaries and not be energetically infiltrated, and the devotion/sealing in of my own energy (via the key protocol applied to the hair and the Nazarite oath) has resulted in a huge supply of creative energy that - since it is no longer siphoned and misdirected - can be applied directly to my own life, family, work, etc. in ways I have never been able to do, resulting in truly miraculous joy, vibracy and unprecedented creativity.

I also have ever increasing amounts of physical strength and stamina and have seen numerous nagging health issues within me resolve completely and nearly effortlessly, in another "coincidence" with this process. I am in no way surprised by this unfolding, since the "bringing home" and sealing/dedicating of our own energy and life force benefits far more than the hair and is really comparable to a "holy grail"/fountain of youth self-sustaining energetic. For me, this is the deepest gift of this method: the ability to reclaim *oneself* and one's own life force - as devoted to the highest good - to then watch the incredible ripple effect that takes places as a result of that reclamation.

As part of this miraculous ripple effect of joy and overflowing vitality, I am now sharing this method with clients who are also beginning to see results. A recent client cites: "There is something magical about Sara Sophia's hair program. Although aesthetically harsh chemically-produced products seem to give a more instant glamour to your hair, these rituals truly work from the inside out. Sealing in aligned energy from the highest good, is the ONLY thing 'out there' that can ever create the inner glow of the sacred divine feminine that brightens this Earth. Thank you Sara Sophia for being a pioneer in this important work to awaken Her back into our lives and this planet."

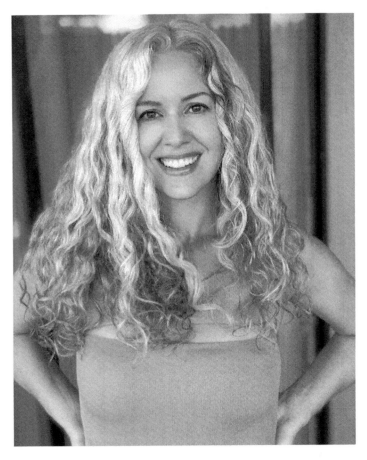

Above: The condition of my hair, as of this writing, October 2018.

My entire family (including my husband, Hanan, and our two children, 10 and 7) has now taken the Nazarite oath, and Hanan is experiencing regrowth from his own male-pattern loss, as he further devotes to this protocol in healing his own hair. This process can take some time for men, as the follicles become damaged/dormant from the male hormones acting upon them and require a bit more to clarify and re-activate. However, Hanan is already seeing an increase in energy and strength, as well as hair regrowth, and I feel strongly this will make a huge difference for him and many other men over time.

I am really excited to offer this method to the world, and am eager to hear how it's working for *you*. I have created an online group for people to share their reflections and results, and would be just as happy to receive messages and testimonials via my website www.sarasophiaeisenman.com as you continue to navigate this unique means of hair regrowth!

If you would like additional support wherever you may find yourself in this journey, please remember to use the additional tools that I've created to benefit and support this process, which can also be found on my website. I am so excited to see what amazing opportunities and community will develop from this as we all continue to grow, and grow beautiful hair, together!

With deepest love always,
Sara Sophia

APPENDIX A: *The Nazarite Oath*

**Original text from the Hebrew bible book of Numbers
(New International Verson, with alternate spelling *Nazirite*)**

6 The Lord said to Moses, 2 "Speak to the Israelites and say to them: 'If a man or woman wants to make a special vow, a vow of dedication to the Lord as a Nazirite, 3 they must abstain from wine and other fermented drink and must not drink vinegar made from wine or other fermented drink. They must not drink grape juice or eat grapes or raisins. 4 As long as they remain under their Nazirite vow, they must not eat anything that comes from the grapevine, not even the seeds or skins.

5 "'During the entire period of their Nazirite vow, no razor may be used on their head. They must be holy until the period of their dedication to the Lord is over; they must let their hair grow long.

6 "'Throughout the period of their dedication to the Lord, the Nazirite must not go near a dead body. 7 Even if their own father or mother or brother or sister dies, they must not make themselves ceremonially unclean on account of them, because

the symbol of their dedication to God is on their head. 8 Throughout the period of their dedication, they are consecrated to the Lord.

9 "'If someone dies suddenly in the Nazirite's presence, thus defiling the hair that symbolizes their dedication, they must shave their head on the seventh day—the day of their cleansing. 10 Then on the eighth day they must bring two doves or two young pigeons to the priest at the entrance to the tent of meeting. 11 The priest is to offer one as a sin offering and the other as a burnt offering to make atonement for the Nazirite because they sinned by being in the presence of the dead body. That same day they are to consecrate their head again. 12 They must rededicate themselves to the Lord for the same period of dedication and must bring a year-old male lamb as a guilt offering. The previous days do not count, because they became defiled during their period of dedication.

13 "'Now this is the law of the Nazirite when the period of their dedication is over. They are to be brought to the entrance to the tent of meeting. 14 There they are to present their offerings to the Lord: a year-old male lamb without defect for a burnt offering, a year-old ewe lamb without defect for a sin offering, a ram without defect for a fellowship offering, 15 together with their grain offerings and drink offerings, and a basket of bread made with the finest flour and without yeast—thick loaves with olive oil mixed in, and thin loaves brushed with olive oil.

16 "'The priest is to present all these before the Lord and make the sin offering and the burnt offering. 17 He is to present the basket of unleavened bread and is to sacrifice the ram as a

fellowship offering to the Lord, together with its grain offering and drink offering.

18 "'Then at the entrance to the tent of meeting, the Nazirite must shave off the hair that symbolizes their dedication. They are to take the hair and put it in the fire that is under the sacrifice of the fellowship offering.

19 "'After the Nazirite has shaved off the hair that symbolizes their dedication, the priest is to place in their hands a boiled shoulder of the ram, and one thick loaf and one thin loaf from the basket, both made without yeast. 20 The priest shall then wave these before the Lord as a wave offering; they are holy and belong to the priest, together with the breast that was waved and the thigh that was presented. After that, the Nazirite may drink wine.

21 "'This is the law of the Nazirite who vows offerings to the Lord in accordance with their dedication, in addition to whatever else they can afford. They must fulfill the vows they have made, according to the law of the Nazirite.'"

The Priestly Blessing

22 The Lord said to Moses, 23 "Tell Aaron and his sons, 'This is how you are to bless the Israelites. Say to them:

24 "'The Lord bless you
    and keep you;
25 the Lord make his face shine on you
    and be gracious to you;
26 the Lord turn his face toward you

and give you peace."'

27 "So they will put my name on the Israelites, and I will bless them."

APPENDIX B: *Supplements and Sources*

(Note: these are just possible online sources to get the following supplements, and there may well be other, less expensive alternatives. That said, I do not recommend using amazon.com for consumable items because they use many different vendors, and it's hard to know the true origins of your items - which I personally find is a problem for safety and quality control. Here, I am offering sources that I know to be mostly reliable/safe, but the reader is of course encouraged to find your own sources, just be sure they are coming from a well-established vendor of which you are truly aware of their quality standards.)

Highly recommended:

Viviscal - available at Target:
https://www.target.com/p/viviscal-hair-growth-supplements-for-women-60ct/-/A-10892786

black currant oil (capsules) - available at Swanson:
https://www.swansonvitamins.com/now-foods-black-currant-oil-500-mg-100-sgels

Great Lakes collagen powder - available at Swanson:
https://www.swansonvitamins.com/great-lakes-beef-gelatin-collagen-hydrolysate-16-oz-454-grams-pwdr

Nordic Naturals fish oil (capsules) - available at Vitamin Shoppe (also, most likely, your local health food store):
https://www.vitaminshoppe.com/p/nordic-naturals-omega-3-1000-mg-60-softgels/ye-1006?
mr:trackingCode=9E175D84-C9E0-E511-80ED-00505694403D&mr:referralID=NA&sourceType=sc&source=SHOP&acqsource=adlucent&utm_source=Shopping&utm_medium=CSE&utm_campaign=Nordic
%20Naturals&utm_content=YE-1006&gclid=EAIaIQobChMIk5_BwrTz3QIV7ZTtCh2ccQuuEAQYAiABEgK0y_D_BwE

Green Pasture fermented cod liver oil/butter oil blend - available from the manufacturer:
https://www.greenpasture.org/public/products/fermentedcodliveroilconcentratedbutteroilblend/

If you are opting for a vegan protocol, I highly recommend:

horsetail/nettles (combined as a tea) - both available at Mountain Rose Herbs:
https://www.mountainroseherbs.com/

Consider also: biotin, copper/zinc (in proper ratio, highly bioavailable forms) - available at most local health food stores

For topical use during the key protocol:

pomegranate oil - available at Mountain Rose Herbs:
https://www.mountainroseherbs.com/products/pomegranate-seed-oil/profile (I recommend the one sourced from the Netherlands)

APPENDIX C: *Topical Hair Product Suggestions: Shampoos, Conditioners, & Styling Products/Oils*

Shampoo/Conditioner:

These are just a few possible recommendations for shampoos and conditioners that would be natural and organic enough to support hair healing. There are likely many others and the reader is encouraged to investigate and explore what works best for them!

Alaffia Everyday Shea shampoo and body wash (found at most health food stores)

Theraneem Organix Scalp Therape shampoo/conditioner - (available at swanson.com)

Desert Essence Coconut shampoo/conditioner - (available at swanson.com)

Tree to Tub Organic Argan Oil shampoo and conditioner - (available at treetotub.com)

Styling Oils and Cremes:

Andalou Naturals 1000 Roses Moroccan beauty oil - my absolute favorite, smells like heaven and contains nourishing oils including pomegranate, argan and more. For use on hair and skin, I carry a bottle of this with me everywhere!

Acure Marula oil - a good go-to basic oil for smoothing and nourishing hair

Acure Moroccan Argan oil - another good basic for hair or skin

(all available at most local health food stores and/or swanson.com)

RESOURCES: *Supplemental Offerings for Implementing & Succeeding in the Nazarite Method*

Additional offerings to support your success with the Nazarite method can be found at:

www.sarasophiaeisenman.com

To book a shamanic journey or find additional information about energetic/shamanic work, as conducted by Sara Sophia's husband Hanan Eisenman:

www.thesacredfemme.com &

www.esseneshamanism.com

Additional reading about Sara Sophia's journey and the philosophy behind Sara Sophia and Hanan's work can be found in the following books:

She is One by Sara Sophia Eisenman
God is with Us by Hanan and Sara Sophia Eisenman

Additional suggested reading:

The Curly Girl: The Handbook by Michele Bender and Lorraine Massey

Resource for those transitioning to natural silver hair:

The Silver Circle on Facebook

That said, I also love me some background. I find having a knowledge of the cultural and historical context of my craft is enriching and powerful. ~~And to~~

The fellow verse & seeker

I created this channel as a space to share about my craft. Not because I want people to do exactly what I do, or because I have all the answers, I don't.

But hopefully to inspire people to create their own path as I have created mine.

warmest blessings

17666992R00055

Printed in Great Britain
by Amazon